MW00583707

Cleaning and Cleaning Validation: A Biotechnology Perspective

Contributors

Roger Brunkow

David Delucia

Shane Haft

John Hyde

John Lindsay

John McEntire

Robert Murphy

Jill Myers

Karen Nichols

Brenda Terranova

Jon Voss

Edward White

PDA

An International Association for Pharmaceutical Science and Technology

7500 Old Georgetown Road, Suite 620, Bethesda, MD 20814 USA

www.pda.org

Editorial Note

The concepts and ideas presented in this book were developed jointly by the members of the PDA Biotechnology Cleaning Validation Subcommittee. The information presented represents the collective understanding and experience of the committee at the time the material was prepared and assembled. The ideas and concepts are not intended to be, nor do they purport to be, specific recommendations or policy setting guidelines of any one company, person, or group or of the PDA.

Further, it should be understood that while every attempt was made to present information pertinent to the biopharmaceutical industry, representation in the committee was limited because of practical and logistical concerns. Consequently, the ideas and concepts cannot possibly represent nor cover all areas of the biotechnology industry.

10 9 8 7 6 5

ISBN: 0-939459-50-7

Contents

Preface

When we first formed the PDA Biotechnology Cleaning Validation Committee in the Spring of 1992 we had no idea that we were getting ourselves involved in such as engrossing project. None of us knew how much personal time would be involved, how many meetings would be involved, how much interest there was in the subject, how many re-writes would be required, how the cleaning industry would change, or how the biotechnology industry itself would change. Fortunately, however, what was even less expected was how rewarding and how much fun we would have.

Our goal was really quite simple: we initially just wanted to get together to talk about the pressing issues of the time—how do we get our multiproduct cleaning validation programs off the ground and our facilities licensed. We soon realized the extent of the interest in the subject and decided to publish a Technical Report. We wanted to publish a useful document, one that people could pick up immediately put to use.

When the outline of the Report was determined, authors were assigned to individual sections and the writing process began. It became apparent very quickly, however, that if the material was to be of practical use, it must be of sufficient detail to cover all aspects of cleaning and cleaning validation. This realization resulted in the decision to turn the Report into a book.

Although our original estimate of two years to completion was stretched to four, the effort has been worthwhile. Lasting friendships have been made. The first PDA book has been published. A complete compilation of the latest trends and practices on the subjects of biotechnology cleaning and cleaning validation is now available sharing the experiences of numerous industry professionals.

In addition to the authors and the companies they work for, many people and organizations are responsible for the successful completion of this work. Fundamental to the success of this work is the PDA, without which the committee itself would never have been formed. Not only was the PDA the central support to this effort, their help was invaluable in the actual editorial and publishing processes.

As the committee Chairperson, I would like to specifically recognize and thank PDA members Ed Fry, James Lyda, Suzanne Stone, Russ Madsen, and Margaret Wanca. Without Ed Fry we would never have been able to negotiate all of the complexities of working as a small group within a larger organization. Ed single-handedly helped prevent us from self destructing during one of our earlier meetings. During the first two years of the effort, James Lyda helped negotiate, prod, and cajole us to complete our work; his tireless energy was encouragement to all of us. Suzanne Stone helped coordinate and organize many of our efforts and served as a friendly liaison between the committee and the PDA home office. In the final two years, when confidence was waning and motivation was weakening, Russ jumped in and helped pull the final publishing effort off. Margaret Wanca arranged to have the book published, and her staff designed its cover.

I would also like to express my personal appreciation to each committee member for their expertise, their time, their excitement, their encouragement, their jokes (Jill especially), their support, and their laughter—without these common elements we surely would never have accomplished this work. I eagerly look forward to our next meeting?

Jon R. Voss
November 1995

About the Authors

Roger Brunkow

Roger Brunkow is an Eli Lilly and Company Engineering Consultant for Biosynthetic Development and Manufacturing. Mr. Brunkow was involved in the design, construction startup, and operation of the first large scale biotech manufacturing facility for Biosynthetic Human Insulin in 1980 and has been or is similarly involved with six additional facilities for CDER and CBER products. He is a member of the American Society of Chemical Engineers, American Society for Mechanical Engineers, and the PDA. He received a BS in Chemical Engineering from the University of Wisconsin in 1967. He has worked for Eli Lilly and Company for 22 years in various engineering and production management positions.

Dave Delucia

Dave Delucia is an Engineering Manager at Creative Ciomolecules, responsible for the design, construction, and operation of a multiproduct, cGMP facility with separate capacity for mammalian cell culture, bacterial fermentation, and associated purification. Mr. Delucia received his MSME from MIT. He is founder and director of the annual ASME course on bioprocess equipment design and an advanced seminar on process development.

Shane Haft

Shane Haft has over eight years' experience in the pharmaceutical and biopharmaceutical industries and specializes in equipment and utility validation. His experience includes project and field validation management, product evaluation, research and development, and microbiology. Mr. Haft has been actively involved with five facility start-up projects, in two of which he managed all validation activities. Presently an independent consultant and president of Rocky Mountain Compliance Specialists, Inc., Bozeman, MT, his past professional positions include Director of Quality Assurance for BioScience Laboratories; Manager of Validation for Synergen, Inc.; Validation Specialist for Mallinckrodt Medical; and Validation Specialist for Skyland Scientific Services, Inc.

John Hyde

John Hyde is president of JM Hyde Consulting, Inc., a firm specializing in design consultation for hygienic processing systems that are CIP cleanable. For nearly two years prior to the formation of JM Hyde Consulting, Inc., Mr. Hyde was Senior Project Engineer with Synergen, a biopharmaceutical research and manufacturing company in Boulder, Colorado. His work at Synergen included design and implementation of hygienic processing systems and the cleaning validation programs for the firm's large scale and clinical manufacturing facilities. From 1982 to 1992, Mr. Hyde was Manager, Process Design, with Seiberling Associates, Inc., an engineering firm specializing in the design of hygienic processing systems and the application of CIP technology. He is currently finishing the manuscript for a book on CIP technology, to be published in the last quarter of 1995. He holds Bachelors degrees in Food Science and Business Administration and a Masters degree in Food Engineering Science from the Ohio State University.

John M. Lindsay

John Lindsay serves as Manager of Quality Assurance Technical Support for Genentech, Inc. Mr. Lindsay has over 22 years' experience in the pharmaceutical and biopharmaceutical industries. He received his MS in Microbiology from Kansas University. Mr. Lindsay is a certified Specialist Microbiologist SM(AAM) by the National Registry of Microbiologists, serves as the chairperson of the Certification of the National Registry of Microbiologists, and is co-author of PDA Technical Report No. 13, "Fundamentals of a Microbiological Environmental Monitoring Program."

Jill A. Myers

Dr. Jill Myers directs the Process Biochemistry Group at Biogen, Inc., which is responsible for the development and refinement of purification methods of recombinant proteins for use in human clinical trials and commercial production. Prior to joining Biogen, she was responsible for the Recovery Process Development Group at Repligen Corp. Dr. Myers received a BS in chemistry from the University of California, Santa Barbara and a PhD in Biochemistry from UCLA and was a Postdoctoral Fellow at Harvard Medical School.

Robert Murphy

Robert Murphy is a Validation Specialist at Amgen, Inc., responsible for the validation of new processes introduced into their licensed multiproduct manufacturing facility. He is an active member of the PhRMA Biotechnology Manufacturing Issues Committee and has made numerous presentations concerning cleaning validation to the PDA, PhRMA, and the FDA. Mr. Murphy received his BS in Biochemistry from the University of Missouri in 1988.

John E. McEntire

Dr. John McEntire holds a BS in Biology from Texas Christian University and an MS and PhD from the University of Houston. Following Postdoctoral studies in cellular immunology at the University of Texas Medical Branch, he was active in purification and characterization of several cell derived lymphokines while a staff scientist at the Cancer Research Center, Columbia, MO. Dr. McEntire became research director of that institution and directed programs in protein chemistry, immunology, environmental carcinogenesis, and clinical immunology. He was co-founder of IMBIC Corporation, a vehicle for commercialization of his patents and properties, which then became a contract research organization. In 1987, he joined Tektagen, Inc., Malvern, PA, as Vice President, where he developed and implemented cGMP laboratories to support biopharmaceutical regulatory testing needs. While at Tektagen, he was recognized for novel approaches to validation of analytical and biological methods. In 1994, he became Vice President of Microbiological Associates, Rockville, MD, where he directs groups responsible for bioanalytical services, biosafety services, lot release, and process validation services.

Karen Nichols

Karen Nichols is the Quality Assurance Manager of Genzyme, Inc. She is responsible for all QA functions including cGMP training, SOPs, batch record control, validation documentation auditing, product release, and investigations. Prior to her association with Genzyme, Ms. Nichols was the Assistant Director, QA, for ImmunoGen, Inc. Currently attending Suffolk University Law School, she received her BA in Biology/Microbiology concentration.

Brenda Terranova

Brenda Terranova is currently a Staff Engineer at Genetics Institute, Inc. She is responsible for managing and executing validation studies on numerous types of equipment and processes. Her area of specialty is cleaning equipment and cleaning validation. In this role, Ms. Terranova has lead multiple efforts in cleaning equipment selection, cleaning process development, and cleaning validation. In previous positions, she has supervised the transfer of technology from Development to Manufacturing, and provided technical support for Manufacturing process operations. She holds a BS in Chemical and Biomedical Engineering from Carnegie Mellon University and an MS in Chemical Engineering from the University of Massachusetts at Amherst.

Jon Voss

Jon Voss is the Senior Manager of Validation for BIOPURE Corporation. Mr. Voss has over eight years' biotechnology experience in the areas of validation, metrology, and automation, serving previously as the Manager of Validation at Amgen, Inc., and the Section Head of Validation and Metrology for Genetics Institute, Inc. Mr. Voss received his BS in Physiology from the University of California at Davis and his MS in Biomedical Engineering from Boston University. He is the Chairperson of the PDA Biotechnology Cleaning Validation Committee and serves as a member of the PDA Software Validation Committee.

Edward K. White

Edward White is Technical Manager, Process Validation, at Connaught Laboratories, Inc., Swiftwater, PA. He has been involved in sterile process validation since 1978 and has been in the startup and validation of sterile filling facilities as well as biotech and traditional pharmaceutical manufacturing facilities. Mr. White has presented papers on validation for ASTM, Pharmaceutical Seminars, Inc., and other organizations. He is an ASQC Certified Quality Engineer and received a BS degree (1975) from the University of North Carolina at Wilmington.

Introduction

Modern biotechnology is a relatively new industry, especially when compared to the much longer lived traditional pharmaceutical industry. Unique issues distinguish certain aspects of the biotechnology industry from the traditional methods of drug manufacture. Factors such as biological containment requirements, product activities in trace quantities, and aseptic processing requirements have required the development of new and alternative approaches to dealing with biopharmaceutical manufacturing technologies.

These differences in drug manufacturing techniques have naturally resulted in the development of sometimes new and different regulatory concerns. Examples of the kinds of regulatory concerns related to cleaning and product changeover can be found in recent regulatory responses obtained from biotechnology companies seeking licensure of their multiproduct facilities:

> Please submit cleaning validation data to support the request for manufacturing of (product X) with another product.

> Please submit SOPs and data to support the removal of residual product and cleaning agents prior to use of the equipment in the manufacture of (product X).

> Will the product-specific assays described in the cross contamination monitoring program be a part of the lot-release specification for the licensed product?

> Please submit a sample of the documentation which would accompany inoculation suite changeover.

> Your procedures for cleaning validation do not address sampling by the swab method. Have you demonstrated (through validation) equivalence between swabbing and the volume of rinse water assayed by TOC? Has swabbing been incorporated into any of your cleaning procedures? If so, please submit your data. If not, please explain why you are not taking samples using this method.

These examples reflect an important regulatory emphasis that dramatically impacts the biotechnology industry. This regulatory emphasis on cleaning is due at least in part to the overall trend towards multiproduct manufacturing in the biotechnology industry.

Biotechnology production is currently performed by a relatively small number of companies that started with a single licensed product and a facility that was dedicated solely to the production of that product. Cleaning concerns were generally limited to providing assurance that lot-to-lot production consistency was achieved. With the maturation of the industry, the need to develop production facilities capable of producing more than one product is being driven by the new products that are being discovered. Cleaning must now address issues of product-to-product isolation.

Although multiproduct manufacturing has been commonplace in the traditional pharmaceutical industry for years, the introduction of multiproduct manufacturing technology to the biopharmaceutical industry is relatively new. As with most industries, the introduction of new technology is initially handled cautiously. This has also been the case with the regulating agencies. In effect, the regulating agencies have challenged the biotechnology industry. On the surface, the challenge seems simple and reasonable enough:

> **Regulatory Agency Challenge** ... prove that you can clean production equipment adequately, such that residues from the production of one product will not carry over and cross-contaminate the next product ...

What seems simple or reasonable in theory can become extremely difficult in reality. Consider the problem. First, one must define cross-contamination, a formidable task in itself. This is especially challenging for biologically derived products in which a contaminant could be any one or more of thousands of organic and/or inorganic residues introduced or derived during the production process. Adding to this problem is the need to be able to detect the contaminant. For biological processes, detection of the desired drug substance can often be a challenge, let alone detection of a specific contaminant.

Assuming contaminant limits can be reasonably set, one must then be capable of demonstrating that the cleaning procedures are "adequate." In theory, verification of adequacy (through validation) for each cleaning procedure requires the demonstration that the cleaning procedure can reliably and effectively remove or reduce a residue to an "acceptable" level. The validation of a cleaning process must take into account all of the assumptions made about the contaminant(s), the ability to detect the contaminant(s), and the processing conditions that would be affected by these assumptions. One can see then why, for the biotechnology industry, the task of validating a multiple product cleaning process is both new and challenging.

This work is intended to serve as a source of practical, technical information for those persons in the biotechnology industry faced with these cleaning and cleaning validation issues. Case studies and/or actual industry examples are used to support the text when and wherever possible. While much of the material contained within this text is equally applicable to non-biopharmaceutical processes, the emphasis has been focused upon the biopharmaceutical manufacturing arena.

In order to help make the text as practical as possible, three major sections were created. Section I provides an in-depth analysis of the design concepts that lead to cleanable equipment. Also covered in the first section are cleaning mechanisms and cleaning systems. This section is particularly useful to those persons faced with the task of designing systems that will be cleaned and also provides the biochemical background of the mechanisms associated with the removal of common biotechnology soils.

Section II focuses on cleaning validation concepts. While the material is equally useful for single product cleaning, emphasis is placed upon multiproduct cleaning validation. Included in this section are general validation principles as they apply to cleaning validation, detailed analysis principles of cleaning process validation, sampling techniques, analytical methods, and acceptance critria. The material in Section II should be useful to anyone responsible for the development of a cleaning validation program.

Section III provides an overview of multiproduct biotechnology manufacturing procedures. Included in this section is an analysis of the risk to benefit scenarios associated with the various forms of product manufacturing. Analysis of changeover programs, equipment considerations, and material transport as they are affected by multiproduct manufacturing strategies is also included.

Recent challenges have been made to the pharmaceutical industry to improve the practicality and added value of their validation programs. It was with these concerns in mind that the representatives of the PDA Biotechnology Cleaning Validation Committee put together this text on the subject of cleaning and cleaning validation. As a committee, we hope that the material contained within will be of practical use to the reader and that it adds value to any existing or newly created programs.

Section I

DESIGN CONCEPTS

Section I provides information that can be used to design a sound and effective cleaning program. Included in this section is a thorough review of equipment design principals, cleaning mechanisms and cleaning systems.

The most important factor in any cleaning program is the equipment being cleaned. Chapter 1, "Process Equipment Design Considerations," provides an analysis of process equipment design principles. Good design of production equipment and associated piping increases the likelihood of successful cleaning. Often an afterthought, a well thought-out design can frequently eliminate costly manual cleaning procedures or reduce cleaning cycle times. The design of processing equipment such that it can be readily cleaned and validated is a demanding process involving the selection of appropriate materials of construction, finishes, and 3-dimensional design. This chapter examines process system design, mechanical design, surface finish and instrumentation concepts. Using specific examples drawn from the biotechnology industry, each aspect of design is examined and demonstrated for applications ranging from bioreactors to chromatography and filling equipment.

The design of a sound, effective cleaning process, whether Clean-in-Place (CIP), Clean-Out-of-Place (COP), or manual requires a basic understanding of the physical and chemical mechanisms of cleaning. Chapter 2, "Cleaning Mechanisms and Strategies," examines the chemistry and physics of biotechnology soils, soil removal processes, cleaning agents and soil-to-surface interactions. Building upon this foundation, the soil-to-surface and cleaning agent interaction is discussed as it relates to automatic cleaning strategies. Cleaning programs for typical biotechnology process equipment are provided that apply the cleaning mechanisms and processes described earlier in the chapter.

An in-depth analysis of automated cleaning systems used in the biopharmaceutical industry is presented in Chapter 3, "Automatic Cleaning Equipment." CIP systems continue to evolve as both the cleaning and the biotechnology industries evolve. This chapter focuses on the principles employed in typical CIP systems including portable, re-use, and eductor assisted single use systems. Instrumentation used in currently employed CIP systems is also covered, emphasizing the aspects critical to effective system design.

1
Process Equipment Design Considerations

Typically, the "cleanability" of process systems and equipment is an afterthought when designing biopharmaceutical facilities. Project teams involved in facilities design, as well as architectural and engineering design firms, often specify individual pieces of equipment without considering how the equipment will be cleaned. Vendors of bioreactors, chromatography columns, ultrafiltration skids, and other processing equipment focus on their own areas of expertise. All of these groups assume that equipment cleaning is the responsibility of the clean-in-place (CIP) system vendor. This approach to equipment design is inefficient and may lead to excessive costs due to energy usage, chemical costs, and validation costs. Relying on the CIP system vendor to ensure that equipment can be cleaned is analogous to relying on the vendor of a clean steam system to ensure that process equipment can be sterilized.

A more efficient approach is to design process systems and equipment so that they can easily be cleaned. Proper equipment design for cleanability can yield significant benefits: cleaning time can be reduced, chemical use and energy costs can be minimized, and the amount of manual cleaning and disassembly required can be reduced. More importantly, cleaning validation will be simplified, and facility start-up will be faster. Proper equipment design for cleanability is especially important for start-up, validation, and approval of multiple use facilities.

This chapter explores some of the most important criteria for design of cleanable process systems and equipment.

PROCESS SYSTEM DESIGN

The single most important consideration in the development of a cleanable process system is the integration of appropriate cleaning technology into the overall process system design at the conceptual and schematic stages of design. This integration can be successfully accomplished only after the needs of one's specific process have been identified and prior to approval of the piping and instrumentation drawings (P&IDs). Understanding the process begins with a process flow analysis, and continues with an analysis of containment requirements and residue properties. Once these elements of the process are understood, one can determine the configuration of both the cleaning and the processing circuits. A major objective at this stage is the development of a process system design in which the cleaning circuits are as simple as possible, the cleaning is easily effected, and the number of circuits is minimized.

Process System Analysis

One of the first steps in designing cleanable processing systems is to conduct a process flow analysis. This analysis consists of the review of process flows, manufacturing methods and procedures, and production schedules. The resulting analysis should include a review of basic unit operations (e.g., media preparation, fermentation, cell processing, filtration) to establish the sequence of steps and any interactions between steps. This information is important to cleaning system design because it is used to determine how the process equipment and its interconnecting piping can be segmented into logical cleaning circuits.

Containment Requirements

One constraint unique to the biopharmaceutical industry is the containment requirements of the process organism and its residues. For instance, if the process organism containment requirements are less stringent (as for GLSP or BL1 organisms), more piping system flow control options are available (such as transfer panels) because of the ability to use "make/break" connections. Conversely, if the process uses an organism with more restrictive containment requirements, the piping system design options may become restricted. For example, waste from a containment restrictive process may have to be inactivated in the processing equipment or sent directly to a biowaste treatment vessel rather than be circulated or sent to drain. These issues can greatly affect the design of the process and its interconnecting piping and cleaning circuit configuration.

Residue Characteristics

The types of in-process residues encountered can also affect cleaning circuit and piping system configurations. Examples include residues that are toxic or that are difficult to keep suspended in cleaning solutions. In these cases, the processing equipment and interconnecting piping in a given cleaning circuit may need to be minimized to prevent deposition on surfaces that do not contact the residue during normal processing operations.

Cleaning and Process Piping Configuration

Once the process flow, containment, and residue characteristics are understood, the processing and cleaning piping configurations should be established. Effective cleaning circuit configuration relies on the process flow analysis described above to determine the sequence and availability of process equipment for cleaning. Once this has been established, the process system can be divided into logical groupings (or circuits) for cleaning based upon equipment and interconnecting piping availability, residue residence times, and similarity of scale and function.

The overall goal of the piping design should be to automatically clean as much of the processing equipment and interconnecting piping as possible while minimizing the total number of cleaning circuits. There are several ways to minimize the number of cleaning circuits, including utilizing process lines as CIP supply/return, combining lines in series in a circuit, and combining lines in parallel in a circuit. A final consideration is the isolation of the dedicated CIP piping from the process piping. This isolation can be accomplished in several ways and it is essential to protect against product contamination from cleaning fluids.

The design of the interconnecting process and cleaning piping as an *integral* system typically yields far superior cleaning results to other piping configurations. An "integral design" refers to a piping system in which as much process piping as possible is used to supply or return cleaning solutions to or from the processing equipment being cleaned. This approach often minimizes the number of cleaning circuits because of the dual usage of process piping for cleaning supply or return. It also can yield a more cleanable design as the number of connection points between the dedicated cleaning and process piping is minimized.

For example, on a bioreactor, the clean steam header may be used to distribute CIP supply. This approach reduces the valve count by eliminating the CIP header, and the cleaning of steam blocks is improved by eliminating dead legs.

To further reduce the number of cleaning circuits, separate process lines may be linked in series during cleaning. However, care must be taken to assure that the CIP supply pump can maintain minimum flow requirements in the largest diameter lines, despite the flow restrictions of the smallest diameter lines.

To reduce cleaning cycle completion time, various sections of the process equipment may be cleaned in parallel. This may require an engineering analysis to verify that the pressure drops in each parallel leg are similar at the required cleaning flow rates. While the engineering analysis method is generally preferred, a method to verify the actual flow rate in each parallel path may be required, as in instances where residues of high viscosity occur.

A final consideration in the design of process piping is that it should be isolated from dedicated cleaning piping in a fail-safe manner. This approach guarantees the integrity of the process piping system as cleaning solutions are prevented from leaking into product containing lines and equipment. Common approaches include removable spool pieces, transfer panels, and special valving arrangements. A transfer panel is an organized way to handle make-break connections or removable spool pieces. If valves are used for isolation they should be arranged in a double-block-and-bleed configuration. That means that there are two valves in series between the process piping and the dedicated CIP piping (this is the double block), and the space between them is vented to the atmosphere during isolation (this is the bleed). Specialized valves are available that provide this function in a compact arrangement.

Regardless of the isolation approach, the isolation should be verified before each cleaning operation to prevent the possibility of a costly product contamination. The verification may be visual or may use electronic/magnetic sensors to verify the proper status of a spool piece or valve.

Case Study 1.1

A new BL3 cell culture process is to be designed that includes media preparation tanks that supply a seed bioreactor and large bioreactor. Bioreactor harvest utilizes a skid mounted filtration system connected to both the bioreactor and a harvest vessel with flexible connections. The equipment is to be designed such that automated cleaning methods can be used (see Figure 1.1).

Analysis of the process flows indicates that media is supplied to the large bioreactor via a 1 1/2" hard piped connection. The seed bioreactor is hard piped to the large bioreactor with a 3/4" line. The large bioreactor has a fixed vertically mounted agitator, a sight glass, four top mounted 2" ports. Since the process is for a BL3 organism, containment will be a major concern. This means that there can be no make/break connections prior to decontamination. This presents some interesting design challenges as it is likely that the media prep vessel, the seed fermentor and the large bioreactor will have to be cleaned separately due to the relative timing of each operation. It is likely that the interconnecting piping will contain a combination of double block and bleed valving and make/break connections so that the system can be cleaned in a contained manner without dead-ends at double block and bleed points.

(Continued on page 8)

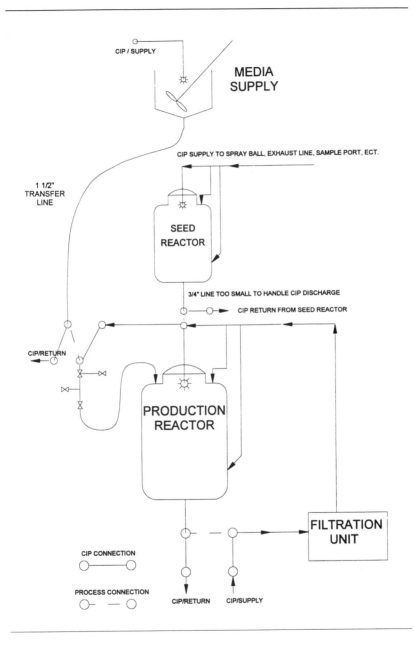

Figure 1.1
Example Case

(Continued from page 6)

The media prep tank and its transfer piping would likely be configured as a single CIP circuit, with the CIP return point adjacent to the large bioreactor. This return point may be a make/break connection as there are no cells in the media prior to fermentation.

The seed bioreactor and its transfer line to the large bioreactor would also likely comprise a single CIP circuit. The 3/4" discharge line might present problems with regard to CIP return from the vessel and should be enlarged. Typically, CIP requirements dictate changing some process line sizes. If the line size cannot be increased, then nitrogen or air top pressure (5-10 psig) may be added to the vessel during CIP, pushing the CIP return fluid out of the vessel. All of the "feeds" into the seed bioreactor should be cleaned in this single CIP cycle, and these may include exhaust piping and filters, gas and/or steam sparging lines, media and/or additive piping, etc. Each of these, while likely small in diameter, will contribute to the overall flow requirements of the circuit and may require automated sequencing as the operation of all at once may result in more flow than can be handled by the 3/4" discharge line. The CIP return point for this cycle will be adjacent to the large bioreactor and, for containment reasons, will be segregated by double block and bleed valving. A make/break connection may also be added upstream of the double block and bleed valving so that they can be thoroughly cleaned later with the large bioreactor.

The large bioreactor, its transfer line to the filtration unit and the filtration unit would likely comprise a single CIP circuit. Even though the discharge piping from this vessel is larger than the seed bioreactor, nitrogen or air top pressure (5-10 psig) may be helpful on the large bioreactor during CIP. As with the seed bioreactor, all of the "feeds" into the large bioreactor should be cleaned in this single CIP cycle, and these may include exhaust piping and filters, gas and/or steam sparging lines, feed tanks, media and/or additive piping, etc. Each of these, while likely small in size, will contribute to the overall flow requirements of the circuit and may require automated sequencing as the operation of all at once may result in more flow than can be handled by the discharge line. Once again, the discharge line should be sized to meet CIP requirements. The CIP return point for this cycle will be near the discharge of the large bioreactor and, for containment reasons, will be segregated by double block and bleed valving. The CIP supply point will also be in the piping near the bottom of the large bioreactor and the cleaning solution flow will be through the filtration unit, into the large bioreactor and to CIP return from the bottom of the large bioreactor.

For more information on cleanable system design, see references 1-3.

DETAILED MECHANICAL DESIGN

The mechanical design phase involves the examination of each piece of equipment with the goal of improving cleaning effectiveness. A detailed mechanical design analysis will serve to determine which surfaces are accessible to CIP, which components must be removed for clean-out-of-place (COP), and how quickly cleaning is accomplished during a CIP cycle. The objective at this stage is to design the process equipment so that dirty surfaces are easily exposed to cleaning fluids.

Mechanical design for cleaning typically encompasses the design of piping, vessels, and components, each of which will be discussed in detail.

Piping

The proper design of process piping is essential to its cleaning by CIP methods. Good piping design for CIP cleaning encompasses several essential principles:

- piping must be sloped continuously to drain points

- the number and length of dead legs should be minimized

- dead legs should be oriented such that they are easily cleanable and drainable

- as much piping as is reasonable within a CIP circuit should be of similar diameter

Three of the four piping design points listed above are often regarded as "general good piping design practice." The last point can be essential in the effective configuration and hydraulic balancing of CIP circuits.

A general "rule" of good hygienic piping design practice is that for the entirety of the process, CIP and SIP piping systems should be installed such that they are completely self draining. Complete drainage is important as it prevents the formation of standing "pools" of liquid that can support the growth of bioburden. Properly sloped piping prevents the formation of condensate "plugs" that can cause cold spots during SIP, and most importantly it allows for the free drainage of all rinsing and washing solutions during CIP, which enhances cleaning efficiency. Typical pitch for a free draining piping system may be as little as 1/16" per foot. Often, larger pitches are specified (1/8" per foot or greater) but these may result in fitting problems, especially where the piping joints are machine welded or attached to piping skids or transfer panels.

Dead legs pose two problems for CIP. First, cleaning fluids must be able to flush out trapped gas pockets in order to wet all of the piping surfaces in the dead leg. Second, fresh cleaning fluids must flush the dead leg to maintain rapid cleaning rates.

The ability to clean a dead leg can be judged by the ratio of its length to its diameter—the "L/D ratio" (see Figure 1.2). The diameter refers to the diameter of the dead leg—not the diameter of the main pipe line. The effective length is measured from the inside wall of the main pipe to the end of the dead leg—for example, at the weir of a diaphragm valve at the end of the dead leg. L/D ratios should be as low as practical. A dead leg with an L/D > 1.5 may be difficult to clean- in-place. Shorter is preferred. Dead leg geometry will affect the minimum required CIP flow rates.

The length of dead legs should be minimized by seeking the shortest tees available, which are those just long enough to accommodate a clamp for a sanitary fitting, approximately 3/4". Minimum branch length tees are readily available for sanitary piping systems. For example, 1 1/2" diameter tees with L/D of 0.6 are available off the shelf. It should be noted that sanitary tees for machine welding are also available with much longer branches (2–4 times the pipe diameter). These should be avoided for circumstances where dead legs are to be minimized. Several fitting manufacturers offer very compact "tee-like" instrument connections that are essentially flush with the inside of the piping in which they are installed. While more expensive than tees, these fittings may be a good choice for applications where any length dead leg is a problem (see Figure 1.3).

Typically, the design of dead legs will determine the minimum liquid velocities required to clean a piping circuit. In a 1" tube, a velocity of only 0.5 feet per second (1 gpm) is required to create the turbulent flow conditions desired for rapid cleaning. However, ten times that velocity may be required to dislodge the gas bubble trapped under a pressure gauge on a vertical tee (see Figure 1.4). Also, longer dead legs require more time and more water to achieve complete rinsing. Minimizing branch lengths will result in more effective cleaning, with potentially lower cleaning solution velocities and reduced rinse and wash times. *An Album of Fluid Motion* by Milton Van Dyke [4] illustrates the effect of geometry on flushing dead legs.

Clear plastic tubing can also be used to visualize the relationship between geometry, flow rates and cleaning. *Conditions for a Pipe to Run Full When Discharging Liquid Into a Space Filled with Gas* by Wallis, Crowley, and Hagi [5] provides a good theoretical discussion of gas and liquid flow in pipes.

Most piping runs have dead legs of some type, whether they are probe penetrations or branches to other runs of pipe. As discussed above, the minimization of the length of dead legs is very important and their orientation is equally important. The preferred orientation of dead legs or branches from process piping is horizontal. Regarding cleaning, a horizontal orientation is best because it offers the best chance of fully flushing the dead leg and removing gas bubbles during the CIP operation (see Figure 1.5). If dead legs must be

L / D = Length of Leg / Inside Diameter of Leg

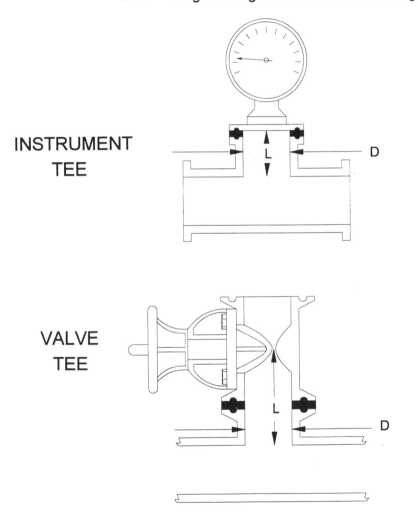

INSTRUMENT
TEE

VALVE
TEE

Figure 1.2
Dead Leg Aspect Ratio

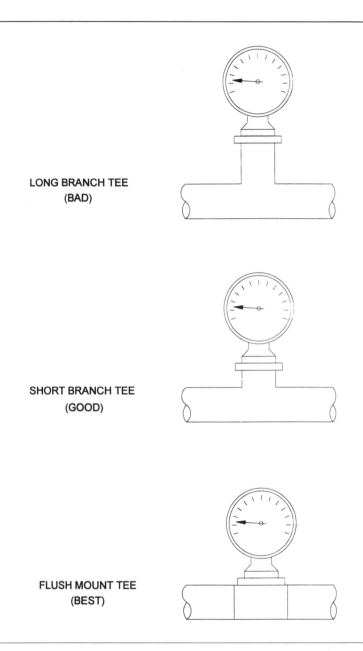

LONG BRANCH TEE
(BAD)

SHORT BRANCH TEE
(GOOD)

FLUSH MOUNT TEE
(BEST)

Figure 1.3
Instrument Tees

IN A 1" DIAMETER TUBE
TURBULENT FLOW PROVIDES
GOOD MASS TRANSFER (CLEANING)
AT 1/2 FT / SEC.

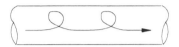

BUT 5 FT/SEC
MAY BE REQUIRED TO ENTRAIN
GAS POCKETS FROM VERTICAL TEES...

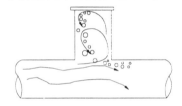

OR TO FLOOD A
DOWNWARD VERTICAL SECTION

(1/2 FT / SEC.)   (5 FT / SEC.)

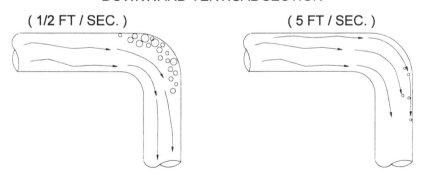

Figure 1.4
Design Details Affect CIP Flow Requirements

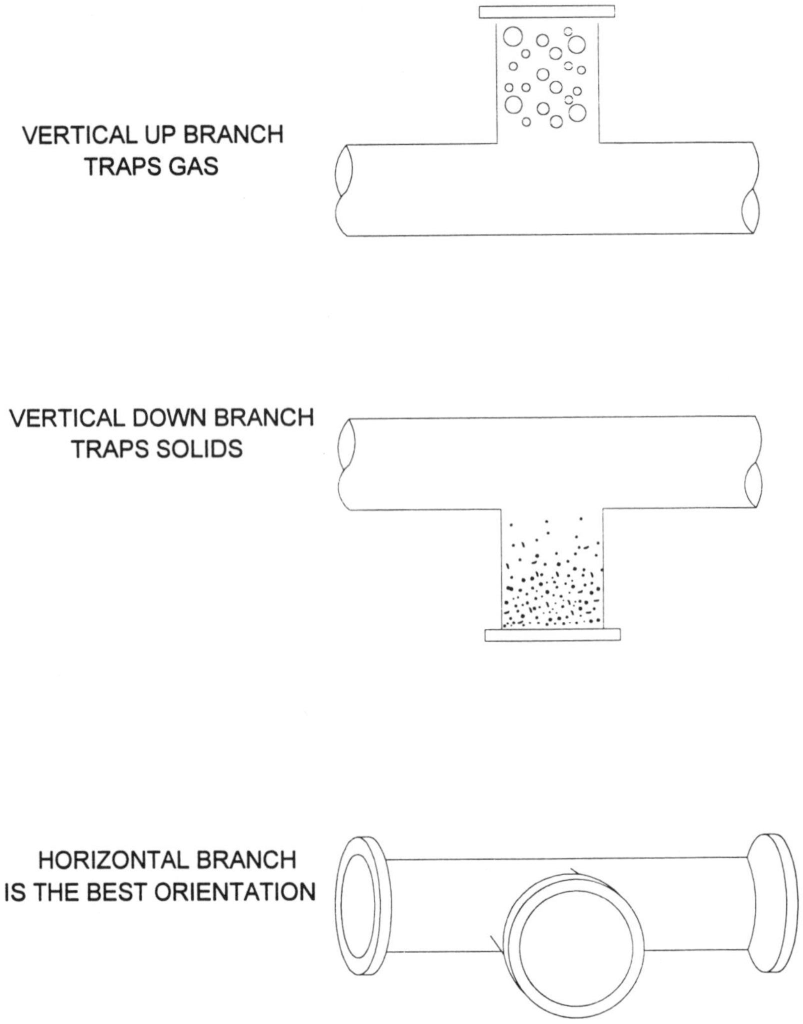

VERTICAL UP BRANCH
TRAPS GAS

VERTICAL DOWN BRANCH
TRAPS SOLIDS

HORIZONTAL BRANCH
IS THE BEST ORIENTATION

Figure 1.5
Dead Leg Orientation

oriented vertically up, then the minimization of their length is of even greater concern because they will be harder to flush due to the problems associated with trapped pockets of gas. A vertically down orientation of dead legs should be avoided. This configuration means that the dead leg would not be fully drainable, presenting problems for both CIP and SIP. If a vertically down configuration cannot be avoided, a "low point drain" is necessary to make the piping system completely drainable.

The sections discussed above the importance of proper piping design: sloping runs of pipe, minimizing dead legs, and orienting dead legs to ensure drainability. As mentioned previously, these are generally good piping design practices. The last topic of discussion in this section concerns the size of piping in CIP circuits. As a general rule, it is best to keep the piping within a given CIP circuit of the same or similar diameter. CIP circuits that contain piping in series of substantially different diameters are often very difficult to balance hydraulically. This is especially true for recirculation based cleaning systems where the supply and return flow rates must be equal for balanced and effective operation.

Where piping sections of substantially different diameter (for example 3/4" and 1 1/2") are cleaned in series, it is often impossible to flow cleaning solutions through the smaller sections at a rate high enough to clean the larger sections. At a CIP solution flow rate of 5 feet per second, the 3/4" piping would require only 4.8 gpm while the 1 1/2" piping would require 23 gpm. This means that the 3/4" sections of piping would have to allow for flow of 23 gpm so that the 1 1/2" piping is adequately cleaned, and this would probably not be possible due to the *very* high pressure drop at 23 gpm in 3/4" piping. Alternatively, these piping sections might be cleaned in parallel rather than in series. However, this alternative also has pitfalls as parallel paths always raise the question of verification of adequate simultaneous flow down each path.

Case Study 1.2

A biotech facility has a buffer preparation area that supplies buffers to several steps in a purification process. These purification steps are in partitioned areas within a common room located 200 feet from the buffer preparation room. The first step requires 1,000 liters of buffer, so the design engineer specifies a transfer pipe of 1" diameter tubing running from buffer prep to purification. The second step requires 200 liters of buffer, so the design engineer specifies a transfer pipe of 3/4" diameter tubing running from buffer prep to purification. Both of these transfer pipes as designed will serve the needs of the process, getting the prepared buffers to the purification area in a timely manner.

(Continued on page 16)

(Continued from page 15)

However, when the CIP engineer steps in (hopefully, before construction) and considers how these two lines will be cleaned, a problem is discovered. This facility has a central CIP system to clean these lines, and it is located in the buffer prep area. Since both of these transfer lines run from buffer prep to purification, the best way to clean them is to create a CIP circuit by connecting them together. This connection means that both lines can be cleaned simultaneously (saving time), and it means that separate CIP return piping will not be necessary (saving money).

After determining that the two lines should make up one CIP circuit, the CIP engineer calculates the pressure drop in this circuit at 10 gpm. Ten gallons/min is chosen because it will result in a velocity of approximately 5 ft/sec in the 1" tubing. With 200 ft of 1" tubing and 200 ft of 3/4" tubing at 10 gpm, the CIP engineer determines the pressure drop will be approximately 80 psi. The CIP engineer then calculates the pressure drop if both runs of pipe were 1" ID. For 400 ft. of 1" tubing at 10 gpm, the pressure drop is approximately 20 psig (4 times lower). The CIP engineer then recommends to the customer that the specified 3/4" tubing be increased to 1" (provided the increase is not a problem for the process) so that a smaller CIP pump might be used, and high pressures during CIP can be avoided. In this example, the additional "hold-up" volume of 1" versus 3/4" piping is not significant. However, for longer runs and larger sizes the increased "hold-up" volume of larger line sizes may be an issue.

This example illustrates the importance of considering CIP during the early design phase of a facility and process piping system. Designing the process piping system such that the line sizes within each CIP circuit are of similar diameters requires an understanding of both the cleaning and processing objectives of the equipment. To be most effective, this input should be provided very early in the detailed mechanical design phase. Bioprocess equipment vendors often do not integrate the best CIP design principles into their designs. Thus, the end user must often serve as the CIP systems engineer who evaluates the cleanability of the proposed equipment, ensuring that all of the parts of the system may be integrated in a manner that facilitates CIP.

In summary, the key detailed piping design criteria that impact the effectiveness of CIP cleaning are sloping runs of piping to drain, minimizing dead legs, orienting dead legs to ensure drainage, and keeping all piping within each CIP circuit of the same or similar diameters. All horizontal runs of pipe should be sloped so that no water heel is left in low points between pipe supports. Water heels may support microbial growth, interfere with SIP operations and lead to ineffective wash and rinsing during CIP. Dead legs can be minimized by seeking the shortest tees available. The length of a tee should be just enough to fit a clamp onto the sanitary fitting, ≤ 3/4." Dead legs should be oriented horizontally (ideally) or vertically up. It is easiest to dislodge air pockets from horizontal dead legs. Vertically down dead legs should be avoided or valved to drain. Finally, as much piping as possible in each CIP circuit should be of the same or similar diameters, as this will result in easier hydraulic balancing, potentially lower operating pressures and more effective CIP cleaning [6].

Vessels

Like piping design, careful design of process vessels can minimize the length of each CIP cycle and the volume of rinse water required to effectively flush the vessel. Furthermore, thoughtful design of a vessel can often allow complete CIP using spray devices and small volumes of water as opposed to flooding the vessel with CIP fluids. Flooding a vessel with CIP fluids is undesirable as it becomes both expensive and time consuming for large vessels. Good vessel design for CIP can be broken down into three areas: nozzles, drains, and inserts.

Nozzles

A nozzle is an opening in the vessel wall on the top or side of the vessel. Technically, the vessel drain is a nozzle, but for the purposes of this discussion it will be treated separately. Examples of typical nozzles include a 2" diameter nozzle on the vessel top for placement of a rupture disk and a 1/2" diameter sample port on the vessel side wall. The design and location of nozzles will determine the ability to deliver cleaning fluids to each nozzle during CIP. Nozzles should be located with CIP access in mind. Typically, the vessel designer will locate the nozzles to accommodate a convenient piping arrangement, without regard to CIP access.

Nozzles on vessels, like dead legs in piping, should be eliminated where possible, and each should be as short and as wide as possible. Nozzles used for instrumentation (e.g., pressure sensors, rupture disks), should be just tall enough to fit a clamp onto the sanitary fitting (approximately 3/4"). The inside opening of nozzles that must pass through insulation should be flared. Insulation is often 1" to 2" thick adding 1" to 2" to the effective length of the nozzle. Nozzles located on the side of a vessel should be sloped so that liquid drains easily either into or away from the vessel (see Figure 1.6).

Nozzles that lead to transfer lines and sample valves are typically not cleaned by spray devices. They are instead typically cleaned by pumping cleaning fluids into the vessel through each such port. Minimizing the number of these ports therefore will help reduce the number of flow paths within CIP circuits.

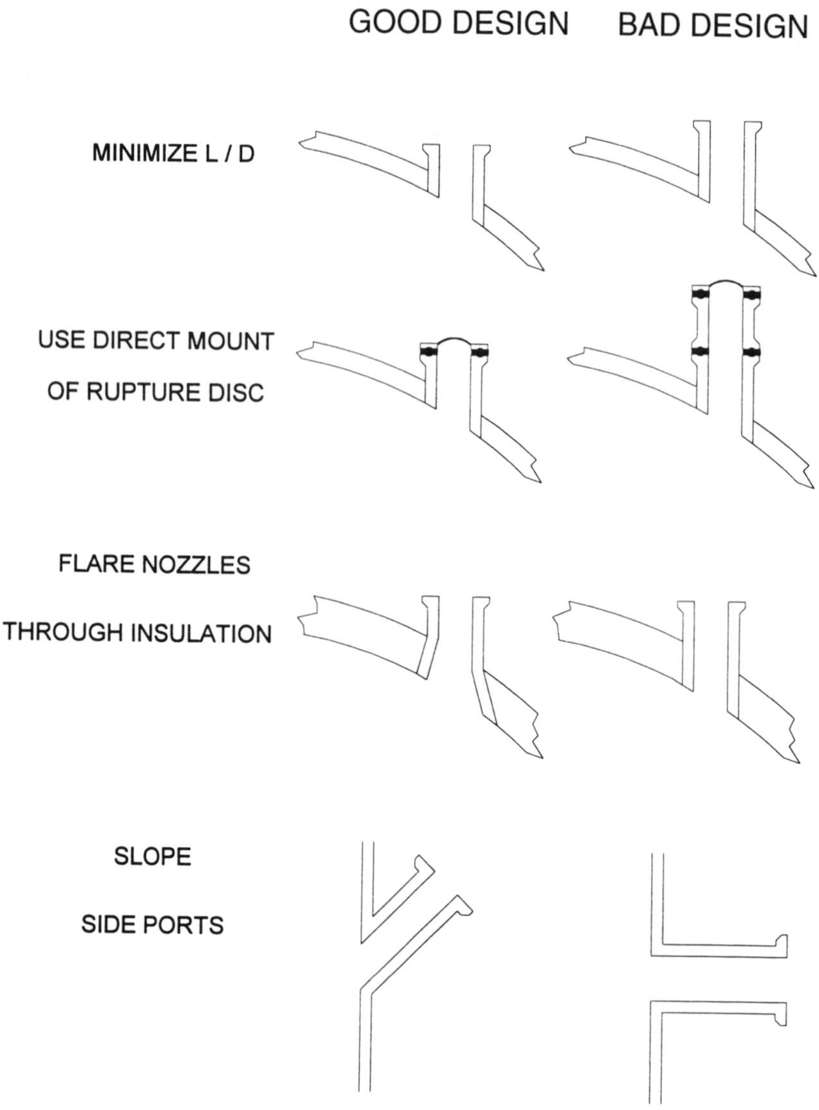

GOOD DESIGN   BAD DESIGN

MINIMIZE L / D

USE DIRECT MOUNT

OF RUPTURE DISC

FLARE NOZZLES

THROUGH INSULATION

SLOPE

SIDE PORTS

Figure 1.6
Nozzle Design for Vessels

Nozzles that accommodate pH and dissolved oxygen sensors should be designed to allow a reliable seal as close as possible to the vessel wall, typically less than 1/2" away. When a nozzle is welded to the vessel wall, the end diameter may become slightly distorted near the weld. To achieve a reliable seal, this distortion should be eliminated by re-boring the nozzle after welding (see Figure 1.7).

Nozzles should be located for the best access to CIP spray. On the vessel top, nozzles should be located close to the spray device. On the upper vessel side wall, nozzles should be located above the spray device. On the lower vessel wall, nozzles such as sensors and sample ports should be virtually flush with the vessel wall to be cleaned by liquid that runs down the vessel wall (see Figure 1.8).

In summary, proper design of nozzles on vessels can aid CIP by ensuring that all vessel internals receive cleaning solution coverage. Generally, nozzles should be small in number, short in length, and fully drainable.

Drains

The vessel drain should be sized to accommodate the maximum fluid flow from all CIP circuits that are run simultaneously, including spray devices and ports that drain to the vessel during CIP. It is a common mistake to size the drain for slow process rates rather than fast CIP rates. If a vessel drain is sized too small, two things can result. First, the high flow rate of cleaning fluid necessary to clean the vessel (see Chapter 3 for details) may not exit the vessel at the same flow rate that it enters. To solve this problem, the vessel might have to be flooded to be cleaned, or cleaning fluid flow could be pulsed to the spray devices, lengthening the CIP cycle.

The second problem with a small vessel drain is that rinse water will accumulate in the vessel and drain slowly at the end of each CIP cycle. Often called a *heel*, this water could leave a film of residue on the side and bottom of the vessel. If existing vessels have drains that are too small to accommodate the continuous supply of CIP rinse water, the rinse may be intermittently pulsed into the vessel. Adequate time must be allowed for complete draining between pulses. Another alternative is to pressurize the vessel during CIP, helping to push the CIP fluids out of the vessel.

Typical drain diameters for several vessel sizes are: 1" for 100 liter vessels, greater than or equal to 1 1/2" for 1,000 liter vessels, and greater than or equal to 2" for 10,000 liter vessels [see 1–3]. In addition to proper size, drains should be recessed to provide complete drainability at the end of a cycle.

Another issue concerning vessel drains is that during CIP of a vessel, a vortex often forms at the vessel drain. The air stream at the center of the vortex is entrained with the liquid and may cause the CIP return pump to become air bound. An air bound pump spins but does not push any liquid and can become

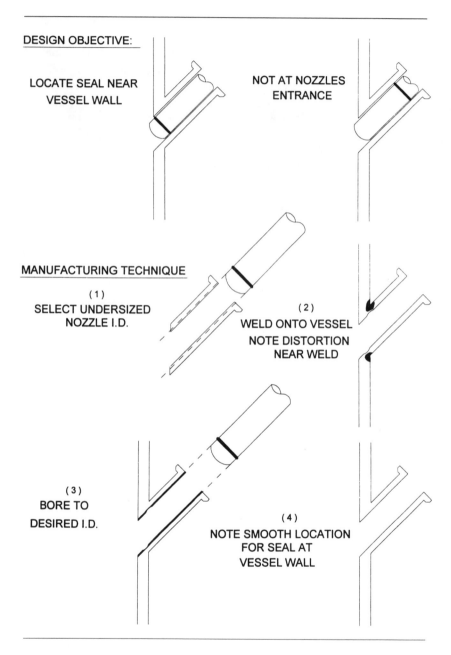

DESIGN OBJECTIVE:

LOCATE SEAL NEAR
VESSEL WALL

NOT AT NOZZLES
ENTRANCE

MANUFACTURING TECHNIQUE

(1)
SELECT UNDERSIZED
NOZZLE I.D.

(2)
WELD ONTO VESSEL
NOTE DISTORTION
NEAR WELD

(3)
BORE TO
DESIRED I.D.

(4)
NOTE SMOOTH LOCATION
FOR SEAL AT
VESSEL WALL

Figure 1.7
Instrument Nozzles

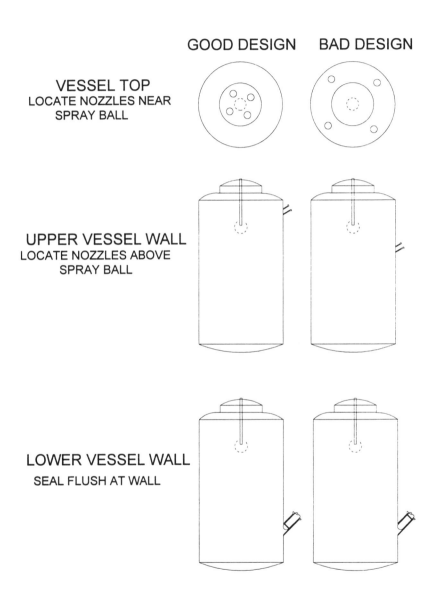

Figure 1.8
Nozzle Location

damaged. To aid in the prevention of vortices, vortex breakers should be installed at the vessel drain. There are two common types of vortex breakers, a flat disk and an "X" of steel (see Figure 1.9). The flat disk is typically 3–4 times the drain diameter and is located 1/2"–1" above the vessel bottom to block air from entering the vortex. The "X" of steel is typically several inches tall and is located at the drain to break up the circular flow that forms the vortex. Both styles of vortex breakers are thoroughly cleaned as CIP fluid flows past them. Even the bottom of the flat disk has passed the surface swabbing tests of cleaning validation.

The line from the vessel drain to the CIP return pump must slope down (see Figure 1.10), which allows air in the line or in the pump to rise back to the vessel. Therefore the elevation of the vessel drain must be specified after the CIP return line and pump are specified. An elevation of 18" to the drain valve discharge is adequate for most situations.

In summary, proper design of vessel drains helps to ensure that the flow rate necessary to clean the vessel can be withdrawn through the drain and that the presence of a heel of water during vessel drainage will be minimized or eliminated. Finally, proper operation of the CIP return pump can be assisted by the presence of a vortex breaker in the vessel and proprer elevation of the vessel drain.

Inserts

An insert is something that protrudes into or is completely contained within a vessel. Examples of typical inserts in bioprocessing applications are baffles, agitators, cooling coils, sparge lines, and sprayballs. Each of these items presents a CIP challenge that can be solved with thoughtful design.

As a general rule, all components and their supports should have rounded edges to encourage free flow of CIP liquids around the corners. Baffles should be welded in place. Welding avoids the cracks and crevices of bolts or pins that can hamper cleaning effectiveness. If the baffles must be removed or changed in the future, they can be cut off and new ones welded to the old support tabs without damaging the vessel wall and without repeating the laborious ASME pressure testing process.

Different agitator designs may require different approaches to CIP (see Figure 1.11). Marine style and flat pitched blade style impellers, typically used in mixing vessels and mammalian cell reactors, can be cleaned by rotating the impeller during CIP. Both the top and bottom sides of each impeller blade will impact spray droplets and surface tension will guide the cleaning fluids around the blades. Traditional Rushton style impellars, typically used in bacterial fermentors, may require CIP spray from below or immersion to clean the bottom side of the large flat disk.

DISC STYLE

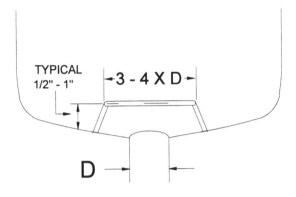

X STYLE

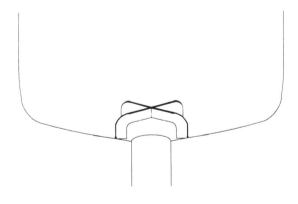

Figure 1.9
Vortex Breaker Design

LOCATE VESSEL DRAIN HIGH ENOUGH TO SLOPE DOWN TO CIP RETURN PUMP

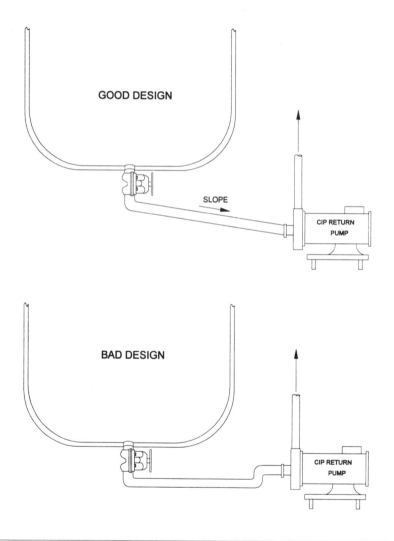

Figure 1.10
Vessel Drain Height

PITCHED BLADE IMPELLERS
CAN BE CLEANED BY
SPRAY FROM ABOVE

(TYPICAL OF GENTLY AGITATED
MAMMALIAN CELL REACTORS)

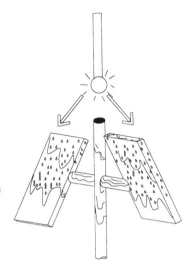

FLAT SUPPORT DISC
MUST BE CLEANED
FROM BELOW

(TYPICAL OF HIGHLY
AGITATED BACTERIAL FERMENTERS)

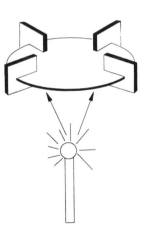

Figure 1.11
Agitator Cleaning

Cooling coils are commonly used inside large bacterial fermentors. To facilitate CIP, the cooling coils should be located far enough from the vessel walls so that spray devices can be positioned between the coils and the vessel wall.

Both bacterial and mammalian culture vessels typically contain sparge lines to supply oxygen to the cells. Sparge lines can typically be CIP cleaned if they are designed to accommodate both the gas flow during processing and the liquid flow during cleaning. Large sparge inserts should also have holes at the low point(s) to ensure full drainage of cleaning liquid. In some cases, the sparger has been used to provide CIP spray to the bottom of a Rushton disk.

Spray Devices

Most large or fixed bioprocessing vessels employ spray devices to effect CIP. During the vessel design stage, the number and location of spray devices must be determined. Spray devices can be mounted permanently in a process vessel, or they can be inserted just for CIP. The use of permanently installed spray devices is recommended to allow repeated process and cleaning cycles without opening the vessel to the environment. Properly designed sprays can be easily sterilized and cleaned-in-place by passing steam or cleaning fluids through them, the same way that a sparger device is sterilized or cleaned in-situ.

Nozzles that will accommodate the insertion of spray devices must be greater than or equal to 3" in diameter to accommodate most commercially available sprayballs. Spray devices for smaller openings can be custom made, if necessary.

Several factors affect the number and location of spray devices necessary in a process vessel. (A detailed discussion of the types of commercially available sprays is provided in Chapter 3.) These factors include the number and type of nozzles and inserts in the vessel. All inserts into the vessel should receive spray coverage. As a result, for a simple vessel, the number of baffles often determines the number of spray devices required in the vessel. Each side of each baffle must be sprayed. All sides of other inserts such as cooling coils and sparge lines must also be sprayed. The number and location of nozzles might also affect the number of spray devices needed. For example, the flow into the vessel from a side–mounted sample port might provide good coverage of a low agitator blade, thereby eliminating a lower spray device.

The relative location of the spray devices, top nozzles and side nozzles should be reviewed before approving vessel drawings for fabrication. After fabrication, the spray coverage can be verified with visual markers and spray test. Some vessel fabricators now offer to execute a spray coverage test at their factories. Common markers used include riboflavin (0.2 gm/l) or a paste made from powdered milk and water. The marker is applied manually and then aspray cycle run. A visual examination of the inside of the vessel will reveal whether all areas were reached by the cleaning fluids (presence of riboflavin is detected with the use of a UV lamp, and the riboflavin must be wet to fluoresce). It is important to run such tests at the expected flow rates and pressures that will be used for cleaning.

In summary, the careful design of inserts into a processing vessel can facilitate CIP. Inserts should be designed to be drainable and to facilitate CIP (e.g., no horizonal surfaces) when possible. Spray devices inserted into vessels should be positioned to provide full coverage of all vessel inserts including baffles, agitators, cooling coils, and sparge lines. Nozzles should be located in relation to the spray devices. Drains should be sized for CIP flow rates. Vortex breakers should be used on drains to minimize the occurrence of an air-bound CIP return pump.

SURFACE FINISH

Once the process system and detailed mechanical design have been completed, the surface finish must be considered. This consideration includes not only the smoothness of the surface but also the way surfaces are welded and the ongoing maintenance of the surface.

There are few empirical studies to demonstrate that high mechanical polish and/or electropolishing are necessary for efficient cleaning [7]. It has become common practice to specify a surface finish of 10–20 microinches roughness average (RA) after electropolishing for wetted process surfaces.

The welding process produces a surface that is typically exposed to process fluids and is often CIP cleaned. As a result, care in welding is important to ensure that a cleanable surface results. Welds should fully penetrate a joint, to fuse both pieces without a crack or crevice between them. Oxygen should be fully purged locally prior to welding. A little oxygen present will cause slight discoloration near the weld. A gross excess of oxygen will cause severe discoloration and bubbling of the surface near the weld. Documented visual inspection of all process welds will detect problems caused by poor fit-up, purging, or welding execution. A record of the amperage and duration of the weld process will not indicate whether fit-up or purging were done properly.

The most commonly used material for bioprocess equipment is 316 stainless steel. The major components of 316 stainless steel are iron, chromium for corrosion resistance, nickel for ductility, and molybdenum for resistance to local chloride attack [8–9]. Low carbon grades (316L) are used for materials that will be welded. If the low carbon grade is not used for welding, then the local area may corrode and become rough and difficult to clean.

The durability and long-term cleanability of a stainless steel surface finish depends on the maintenance of the passive oxide layer. Maintaining this layer means avoiding design and operating practices which foster corrosion. Continuously hot process surfaces are of specific concern because the heat can cause precipitation of process fluid components onto metal surfaces. If not cleaned, this impervious layer of dirt can lead to severe crevice corrosion [10].

A tough chromium oxide layer on the surface of stainless steel resists corrosion and is the primary reason for the "stainless" appearance. This passive oxide layer forms the moment that stainless steel is exposed to the atmosphere. Strong, hot acids are not required to create this passive film. The passive layer is "self-replenishing" in the presence of air or oxidizing fluids. This passive layer will reform when exposed to the atmosphere after welding, machining, or scratching the stainless surface. However, the chromium oxide layer may break down under impervious layers of dirt. Therefore, routine cleaning is the key to maintaining the corrosion resistance of the process equipment.

The traditional process called *passivation* is actually a good, thorough cleaning performed after fabrication is complete, just prior to putting the process equipment into service. It is no coincidence that the typical passivation procedure mimics the typical CIP procedure: caustic to dissolve grease and oils, acid to dissolve other deposits, and plenty of rinsing [11]. A clean stainless steel surface is a passive surface. Chemically assisted passivation or re-passivation is typically not necessary if the surface is kept clean.

In summary, surface finish is an important element in process equipment design. A good surface finish aids cleanability and ensures long life for the process equipment. Specifying a durable surface finish includes the consideration of material specifications, welding, cleaning and the identification and ongoing maintenance of areas prone to corrosion.

COMPONENT SELECTION

Once the process system design, detailed mechanical design, and surface finish selection are completed, the system components must be selected. These components include such things as seals, valves, pumps, sensors, filter housings and filter materials, resins, chromatography columns, filling equipment, biowaste systems and centrifuge. Two sets of generalized criteria are often used to help select proper components for bioprocessing operations. These include checking to make sure that the components themselves are designed to be thoroughly and efficiently cleaned in place, and that the components are specified to handle the flow rates, temperatures, and chemical compatibility required for cleaning conditions.

Seals

Static seals such as O-rings and sanitary fittings have no moving parts. Static seals should be designed with no metal-to-metal contact between the process fluid and the elastomer seal. For example, a traditional O-ring gland does have metal-to-metal contact between the process fluid and the O-ring. That metal-to-metal barrier is likely to prevent complete SIP and CIP up to the O-ring itself (see Figure 1.12).

Static seals should be selected that minimize extrusion of the elastomer gasket into the process stream. During SIP, elastomer gaskets and O-rings will thermally expand about ten times more than the steel around them. The seal geometry should be designed to accommodate this thermal expansion. Often, fittings originally designed for the dairy industry do not accommodate the thermal expansion of the gasket. The common result is that the gasket expands

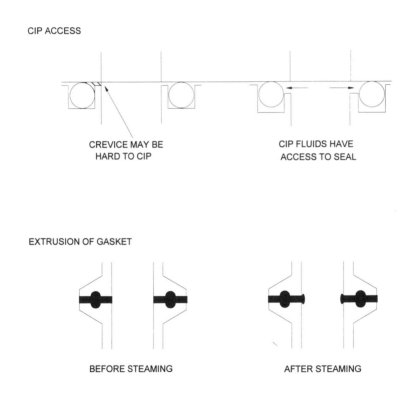

CIP ACCESS

CREVICE MAY BE
HARD TO CIP

CIP FLUIDS HAVE
ACCESS TO SEAL

EXTRUSION OF GASKET

BEFORE STEAMING

AFTER STEAMING

Figure 1.12
Static Seal Design

during SIP and extrudes radially inward, into the process stream. After SIP, when the elastomer has cooled, it remains protruded like a champagne cork that does not go back into the bottle. The net result is a gasket that protrudes into the process stream during processing and subsequent CIP. Common sanitary style gaskets for 1/2" diameter tubing can swell so much that they severely restrict flow through the tubing. On larger lines the swelling may not be significant.

Valves

The most commonly used valves in process piping systems for biopharmaceutical manufacturing are diaphragm valves. This is because they are easily CIP cleanable and provide complete containment of in-process materials. Diaphragm valves are limited in the ways they may be installed for free drainage; they sometimes are prone to leakage and they have a relatively high pressure drop as compared with other types of valves. For situations where complete containment is not required, "plunger-type" compression valves of hygienic design may be used. These have several advantages over diaphragm valves regarding installation and operation but they do not provide complete containment. Areas where "plunger-type" compression valves may be used include CIP distribution piping and non-sterile parts of a given process. Several manufacturers of hygienic compression valves offer versions that are internally leak protected, thus eliminating the need for "double block and bleed" arrangements in configurations such as those for the isolation of process and CIP piping.

Ball and butterfly valves are also commonly used in biopharmaceutical manufacturing facilities. However, because of their design neither of these types of valves is CIP cleanable, and they should *not* be used in process or CIP piping systems. Ball and butterfly valves may be well suited for certain utilities such as process air, chilled water, clean steam, etc., but their use should be discouraged in piping systems where they will contact in-process materials or cleaning solutions.

Pumps

Several types of CIP cleanable pumps are commonly used in biopharmaceutical manufacturing processes. These include centrifugal, rotary lobe, peristaltic and diaphragm pumps, of which all but the centrifugal pump provide positive displacement. Centrifugal pumps are commonly used for applications where the process fluid is not shear sensitive and relatively high flow rates are required. In biopharmaceutical manufacturing processes, this may include the transfer of materials such as media, buffers, water and/or CIP solutions.

Positive displacement pumps are more commonly used in biopharmaceutical manufacturing processes where one or more of the following criteria apply:

- process fluid is shear sensitive

- flow rates are relatively low

- precise flow rate and/or pressure control is required

Pumps used in chromatography systems often include rotary lobe, diaphragm, peristaltic, and cogwheel. Peristaltic pumps offer the advantage of easy changing of tubing. Rotary lobe pumps may be CIP cleanable or readily opened for cleaning. Diaphragm pumps, which are also used in production chromatography, offer the advantage of no fluid contact with a rotating mechanical seal. Challenge studies with American Type Culture Collection Water for Injection (WFI) test microorganisms have shown that these pumps are readily sanitized. However, diaphragm pumps can generate significant pulsations during operation, which can have undesirable effects on the equipment and piping downstream. Pulsation can be reduced by throttling the pneumatic air supply.

Diaphragm and peristaltic pumps avoid the complexity of mechanical seals; however they may not be suited for SIP or high pressure operation. Standard models may require additional diaphragm support for high temperatures or high pressure applications. Rotary lobe pumps are often used for this application although centrifugal pumps may also be used. If a rotary lobe pump is used, it should *not* be specified with an internal pressure relief valve as these are *not* CIP cleanable. The temperature conditions under which the rotary lobe pump operates should be well understood as the lobes may require additional clearance for high temperature applications. Also, while all hygienically designed centrifugal pumps are CIP cleanable, it is important to note that some hygienically designed rotary lobe pumps are not.

In-Line Instrumentation

In-line instruments or sensors are necessary components for automated processes. For ease of cleaning, sensors should be chosen that directly mount onto vessel nozzles or piping tees with minimum dead leg distances. Also, the instruments should be of a cleanable design and constructed to similar standards as those for process equipment and piping. Some specific examples are given below (see Figure 1.13).

Pressure Gauges: Sanitary diaphragm-style pressure gauges should be used when possible, as they are very cleanable. When pressure gauges are installed in process piping, full diameter tees

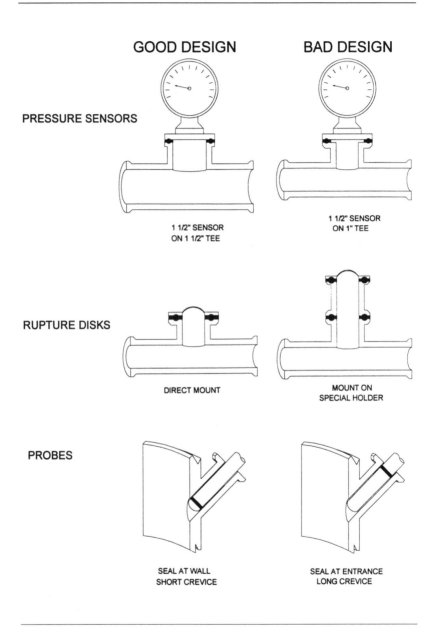

Figure 1.13
Instrumentation

should be used. For example, a 1 1/2" diaphragm pressure gauge should not be installed on a 1" tee even though it does fit the same sanitary connection, there would be a 1/4" annular crevice at the seal. In this case, the main line should be enlarged to 1 1/2" diameter and a 1 1/2" diameter tee should be used, or a smaller gauge may be used. Sanitary diaphragm-style pressure gauges are available in sizes as small as 3/4" diameter for small lines

Pressure Relief: Rupture disks are often the preferred choice over pressure relief valves, because spring-loaded pressure relief valves can become lodged open by debris. This in turn may cause vessel integrity and cleaning problems. The use of a rupture disk followed by a pressure relief valve should be avoided as the relief valve can potentially mask a pin hole leak in the rupture disk.

Rupture Disks: Rupture disks should be chosen to mount directly onto piping tees or vessel nozzles to minimize dead legs. If possible, a rupture disk that mounts directly onto a sanitary fitting without an intermediate spacer is preferred as this configuration minimizes the dead leg between the rupture disk and piping or vessel dome.

pH & DO$_2$ Probes: Dissolved oxygen and pH probes should be sealed as close to process fluids as possible. This may require the re-boring of the inside of the probe holder *after* it is welded into a process line or vessel. This provides good dimensional control for an O-ring seal as close as possible to process fluids. Re–boring of the probe holder is occasionally required to correct distortions caused by welding.

Level Indicators: Several types of CIP cleanable level indicators are available including process fluid contacting and non-contacting devices. Ultra-sonic level sensors and load cells are each of the non-contacting variety, while differential pressure (DP) cells, point and continuous probes, floats and bubblers comprise the commonly used contacting types. Any of these types of devices can be applied in such a way that they can be effectively CIP cleaned. DP cells must be installed such that they are flush with the inside of the vessel sidewall or bottom dish, and probes and floats must be installed such that they may be effectively spray cleaned. Foaming can present difficulties in the operation of several of the devices including ultrasonics and point and continuous probes. When float-type devices are used, complete cleanability can be an issue.

Ultraviolet (UV): Ultraviolet flow-through cells should be sized carefully. Often the short path length required to give good sensitivity is not large enough to allow for CIP flow rates. Large diameter in-line sensors are available where the UV detection components protrude into the process stream, allowing a small path length without fully restricting the fluid flow. The use of stream splitters can result in clogging problems and should be considered carefully.

Air Detection: Where available, non-invasive monitors for air detection are recommended. Detectors are available that clip onto translucent small diameter tubing. For larger systems, infrared path detectors can be used on bubble traps to determine when the liquid level in the trap drops below the desired level.

Temperature: Many types of hygienically designed temperature sensors are available. These include invasive and non-invasive designs. Thermal wells that are welded directly into vessels or piping are often used as they are relatively non-invasive and do not require a seal. Temperature sensors that attach to the outside of vessels or piping are also non-invasive but are often less responsive than those that contact process fluids directly. As with other in-line instruments, temperature sensors should be installed according to good hygienic practices, observing criteria such as minimizing dead legs and eliminating crevices and recesses.

Conductivity: There are several types of hygienically designed conductivity probes in common use for biopharmaceutical processes. These are typically the electrodeless type and mount into tees in the piping system. The most common concern with these instruments in terms of cleaning is that they may restrict CIP flow, especially in very small piping.

Filter Materials

The chemical and physical properties of membrane materials often dictate the cleaning methods and agents chosen for microfiltration (MF) and ultrafiltration (UF) equipment. Many MF and UF filter materials have temperature and pressure constraints and some are incompatible with cleaning agents such as sodium hydroxide (NaOH) and surfactants. In any case, the cleaning cycle must be designed such that the membrane materials are not physically or chemically degraded by the cleaning process. In practice, this may require that cleaning not be done using solutions provided by a CIP system due to pressure, flow rate and temperature concerns. With regard to cleaning agent selection, it may be necessary to "clean" the membrane with a very mild detergent, followed by sanitation with sodium hypochlorite or bleach. While bleach alone is not a very effective cleaning agent, it has good sanitizing properties and limited functionality in the degradation of residues.

Resins

If systems containing resins are to be cleaned-in-place, compatibility of the resin with the cleaning agents should be examined. Some chromatography resins are very compatible with commonly used cleaning agents such as sodium hydroxide. In these cases, sodium hydroxide (or some other strong cleaning agent) may be an integral component of the column's regeneration solution, and the resin is cleaned as it is regenerated [12]. Other chromatography resins, such as those containing protein ligands, are not compatible with sodium hydroxide. It is not uncommon for the resin and/or the column to be incompatible with the cleaning solutions provided by typical CIP systems. This may be due to concerns about the potentially damaging effects of cleaning agents, solution flow rates, pressures and/or temperatures. To address these concerns, special consideration is often given to the design of the feed and discharge piping such that the chromatography column can be isolated during the cleaning of the rest of the chromatography system, thus protecting the resin from potentially damaging cleaning chemicals.

Chromatography Columns

Cleaning of chromatography columns depends upon internal configurations that provide good flow distribution and a minimum number of crevices and dead spaces. Columns requiring the bed support to be attached to the flow distributor with bolts through the bed support can have poor flow distribution along this outer edge, potentially resulting in inadequate cleaning in these areas [13–14]. In addition, columns typically have a gasket that seals the bed support to the walls of the column tube. If this gasket is located too far above the bottom of the top flow distributor, a dead space of resin around the edge of the top flow adapter can result.

Filling Equipment

Time/pressure fillers typically can be cleaned-in-place, while piston and diaphragm fillers typically cannot be cleaned-in-place. Choice of final fill equipment is based on several factors, including equipment cost, ease of changeover, product hold-up volumes, and filling factors, as well as cleanability. Specific considerations in the design of CIP cleanable filling equipment include the location, configuration and size of surge tanks in the filling line, the design and installation of instrumentation (such as level probes in the surge tank) to ensure their compatibility with CIP, and the design of the filling manifold such that there are adequate flows of cleaning solutions through filling needles and the filling line. Specific considerations for filling equipment that must be cleaned-out-of-place include design for easy disassembly and re-assembly under aseptic conditions and a design that allows for easy replacement of elastomers during product changeovers.

Biowaste Systems

The general design guidelines presented earlier also apply to biowaste systems. The biowaste system should be fully cleanable because the build-up of precipitated solids will impede steam decontamination. Periodic cleaning is also necessary to maintain the passive oxide layer of the stainless steel. Without periodic cleaning, the combination of precipitated solids, high chloride concentrations, and high temperatures may cause crevice corrosion.

Centrifuges

Two types of centrifuges are widely used in biopharmaceutical processes. These include tubular-bowl and disk centrifuges [15]. Because of the requirement of bowl removal for solids recovery, tubular-bowl centrifuges are most often not CIP cleaned in their entirety. The bowl is nearly always manually cleaned or COP'd, and the rest of the machine is typically manually cleaned, although design modifications may make CIP cleaning possible. As with other manually cleaned equipment, the design of the equipment should be such that complete cleaning is possible. These types of design criteria include items such as easy disassembly and reassembly, radiused corners, cleanable surface finishes, accessibility of all product contact areas, and others mentioned above.

Continuously de-sludging disk centrifuges (including nozzle discharge machines), if designed appropriately, can be CIP cleaned relatively easily. Cleaning typically involves the recirculation of cleaning solutions through the machine in the same manner as the product feed and discharge. The cleaning flow rate is often higher than that for the product, although this may vary. The materials discharged from the bowl during cleaning may be sent to drain or recirculated, depending upon the nature of the residue. The proper timing of the bowl opening and the sequencing of the CIP valving on the machine are important parameters in the CIP cleaning process.

Disk centrifuges that are not continuously de-sludging are typically not CIP cleanable as the heavier residues will collect in the bowl and not be easily flushed from the machine. Because of the requirement of bowl removal for solids recovery, these types of disk centrifuges are most often not CIP cleaned in their entirety. The bowl is nearly always manually cleaned or COP'd, and the rest of the machine is typically manually cleaned. The same comments apply to the manually cleaned disk centrifuge.

Filter Housings

In-line filtration is a very commonly applied unit operation in biopharmaceutical manufacturing processes. The housings used for filtration are often CIP cleaned (cartridges removed) with their interconnecting process piping. This can be done effectively in some cases and can present significant cleaning problems in others. Where possible, the "flow through" or "in-line" type housings should be used as they provide better flow characteristics for cleaning than do the "tee-style" housings (see Figure 1.14). This is because tee-style devices are configured for fluid entry and exit from the same end of the housing, and could result in significant "short circuiting" of flow and potentially insufficient solution contact velocity and mixing. By contrast, the in-line housings represent no more than an enlargement in the piping and thus can be effectively contacted by cleaning solutions. For either the in-line or tee-type housings, cleaning will be more difficult as the diameter difference between the piping and the housing increases. That is, a "1-round" housing with 1" feed and discharge piping should be easier to clean than a "9-round" housing with 2" feed and discharge piping because the diameter difference is the smallest for the 1" housing and its piping. The main advantage of the tee-type housings is that their cartridges can often be more easily replaced than those in-line housings. However, for purposes of cleaning, the in-line housings are most often the best choice as they allow for the best flow characteristics for the cleaning solutions.

   In summary, the selection of cleanable components is another important factor in process system design. Good components will have minimal crevices, be fully drainable, and be compatible with CIP conditions.

SUMMARY

The design of process equipment for effective cleaning involves the integration of process system design, mechanical design, surface finish and component selection. Each of these areas are important in the overall design process and should be considered early on in the equipment design process.

IN LINE STYLE

IN VERTICAL ORIENTATION
CLEANS IN PLACE

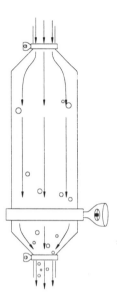

TEE STYLE

TRAPS GAS

OFFERS SHORT-CIRCUIT
PATH FOR LIQUID

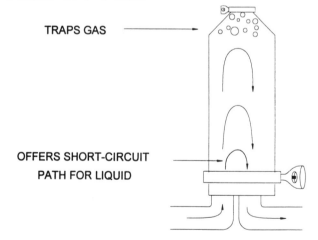

Figure 1.14
Filter Housings

REFERENCES

1. Seiberling, Dale, Notes from ISPE CIP Course, San Diego, CA, February 12–14, 1992.

2. Seiberling, D.A., "Clean-in-Place/Sterilize-in-Place (CIP/SIP)" in *Aseptic Pharmaceutical Manufacturing,* (W.P. Olson and M.J. Groves), Interpharm Press, Inc., Prairie View, IL, 1987, Chapter 11, p. 247.

3. Seiberling, D.A., "Clean-in-Place & Sterilize-in-Place Applications in the Parenteral Solutions Process," *Pharmaceutical Engineering,* Vol. 6, No. 6, 1986, pp 30–35.

4. Van Dyke, Milton, *An Album of Fluid Motion*, The Parabolic Press, Stanford, CA, 1982, p 15.

5. Wallis, G.B., Crowley, C.J., Hagi, Y., "Conditions for a Pipe to Run Full When Discharging Liquid into a Space Filled with Gas," *Journal of Fluids Engineering*, Vol. 99, June 1977, pp 5–413.

6. Green, B., Bioreactor Design Workshop Notes, ASME Bioprocess Equipment Design Course, Charlottesville, VA, October 1992.

7. Villafranca, J. and Zambrano, E.M., "Optimization of Cleanability," *Pharmaceutical Engineering*, Vol. 5, No. 6, November 1985.

8. Tuthill, A.H., *Guidelines for the Welded Fabrication of Nickel-Containing Stainless Steels for Corrosion Resistant Services*, A Nickel Development Institute Reference Book, Series No: 11 0007.

9. Tuthill, A.H., *Guidelines for Selection of Nickel Stainless Steel for Marine Environments, Natural Waters and Brines,* A Nickel Development Institute Reference Book, Series No: 11 003, 1987.

10. Menon, Gopi R., "Rouge and Its Removal from High-Purity Water Systems."

11. Tuthill, Arthur H., Avery, Richard E., "Specifying Stainless Steel Surface Treatments," *Advanced Materials & Processes*, December 1992, pp 34–38.

12. *Sanitizing BioProcess Chromatography Systems with Sodium Hydroxide,* Technical Note 207, Pharmacia Biotech, Piscataway, NJ.

13. Johansson, H., Ostling, M., Sofer, G., Wahlstrom, H., and Low, D., *Chromatographic Equipment for Large-Scale Protein and Purification in Downstream processes: Equipment and Techniques,* Mizrahi, A. ed., Alan R. Liss, Inc., New York 1988, pp 128–154.

14. Sofer, G.S., and Nystrom, L.E., *Process Chromatography: A Guide to Validation*, Academic Press, London, 1991.

15. Mahar, J.T., "Scale-Up and Validation of Sedimentation Centrifuges, Part 1: Scale-Up," *BioPharm*, 6(7), September 1993, pp 42–51.

2

Cleaning Mechanisms
and Strategies

The repeatable, reliable and effective cleaning of biopharmaceutical equipment often depends upon many factors. These include the design and selection of processing equipment and interconnecting piping such that it can be effectively cleaned, an understanding of the chemical and physical properties of the residues to be removed, an understanding of the processes involved in cleaning and the cleaning agents that facilitate these mechanisms, and a clear comprehension of factors affecting cleaning efficiency and their application to specific systems and cycles.

The materials covered in this chapter are intended to address the factors noted above and to review criteria for selection of cleaning strategies appropriate for the equipment to be cleaned and the residues to be removed. Cleaning sequences typical for biopharmaceutical processes are reviewed for processing vessels, equipment and interconnecting piping, membrane filtration equipment, and chromatography systems. Manual cleaning and its validation and/or qualification are also briefly discussed.

CLEANING MECHANISMS AND AGENTS

The selection of appropriate cleaning agents is critical to the success of the application of automatic cleaning methods. A good understanding of the chemical and physical properties of the soils (or residues) to be removed and of the interactions between the residues and the surfaces to which they may be adhered is essential. It is also important to understand how soluble or suspendable the residues will be in the cleaning solution(s) once they have been removed from the surfaces so that they are not re-deposited. The following is a review of typical biopharmaceutical soils, commonly used cleaning mechanisms and agents and their application in the removal and suspension of residues.

Typical Biopharmaceutical Residues

Because many biopharmaceutical products are proteinaceous and their manufacture involves media and buffer preparation, cell growth, cell harvest and processing, product purification, and other steps, biopharmaceutical residues are often composed of proteins, lipids, simple and complex sugars, and salts. Also, because many biopharmaceutical processes require decontamination with steam prior to cleaning, heat denatured residues are a common challenge.

Proteinaceous residue removal can be difficult due to denaturation, insolubility, foaming and other factors. The removal of lipid, sugar and salt residues is often less difficult. When planning for and executing a cleaning program, it is important that there is a good understanding of which of these residue components is present in each processing step such that the cleaning mechanisms and agents can be chosen appropriately. For instance, if the major component of a residue is a protein which is easily degraded and solubilized by acid, it would make little sense to use an alkaline cleaning agent for its removal. However, if at a different step within the process the major residue is comprised of lipids and sugars, an alkaline cleaner might be the best choice. Thus, the cleaning cycle steps and cleaning agents should be chosen based upon the most effective mechanism(s) for removal of the residue specific to that process step and equipment.

Mechanisms Involved in Residue Removal

Several general mechanisms, or processes, of residue removal are commonly employed in the automatic cleaning of biopharmaceutical processing equipment. Ideally, these are matched to the residues and their interactions with surfaces in the development of a cleaning regimen that is reliable and reproducible. The following section describes mechanisms often applicable to the removal of biopharmaceutical residues.

Dissolving

This refers to the direct solubility, without significant chemical degradation, of residues in water or cleaning solution. Examples of water soluble residues include non-heat treated simple sugars, short chain alcohols and monovalent salts. Polyvalent salts are also typically dissolved, but often in acidified solutions. Dissolving is the simplest process of those commonly used in automatic cleaning and therefore the mechanism of choice, if possible.

Saponifying

This process specifically involves the chemical degradation of lipids, which are not freely soluble in aqueous solutions. Saponification is most often accomplished by a hydration reaction where free hydroxide breaks the ester bonds between the fatty acids and glycerol of tri-glycerides, resulting in free fatty acids and glycerol, which are each soluble in aqueous solutions. Heat treated lipid residues are often harder to remove than non-heat treated residues due to polymerization. Saponification is important in the removal of biopharmaceutical residues because lipids are nearly always present in some phase of the process, especially in areas involving cell growth and disruption.

Peptizing

This refers to the degradation and dispersion of proteinaceous residues. Peptizing typically involves the cleavage of protein residues into smaller peptide chains which are soluble in aqueous solutions. Depending upon the physical and chemical properties of the specific protein residue (such as pK values), peptizing can be accomplished by alkaline, chlorinated alkaline, enzymatic, or acidic cleaning solutions. Heat treated proteinaceous residues are typically harder to remove than non-heat treated residues due to denaturation, which can result in residues that are highly insoluble and strongly bonded to equipment surfaces. Peptizing is an important mechanism in the removal of biopharmaceutical residues as proteins are nearly always present in the process, and they often comprise the final product.

Wetting

Because residues are often adhered, or bonded, to equipment surfaces, and because many of these residues are hydrophobic to some degree, it is difficult for cleaning solutions of moderate to high ionic strengths to penetrate and degrade them. Wetting is a process that involves the lowering of the surface tension of the cleaning solution and this allows it to better penetrate residues that are adhered to equipment surfaces. Wetting agents, or surfactants, are often used in relatively small amounts and they can substantially reduce the quantities of cleaning agent (alkali or acid) required for residue removal. Wetting is an important mechanism in the removal of biopharmaceutical residues as many are hydrophobic and strongly adhered to equipment surfaces.

Emulsifying, Dispersing, and Suspending

Once residues have been removed, they can either stay dispersed in the cleaning solution or precipitate and be re-deposited on equipment surfaces. This cycle of removal and re-deposition is inefficient and will likely lead to incomplete residue removal. Emulsifying and suspending agents are often used to keep residues from precipitating by providing hydrophobic groups onto which hydrophobic areas of residues can associate, thus preventing them from associating with other residues and forming larger particles which are likely to leave solution. The emulsifying and suspending agents also typically have hydrophilic groups which keep them soluble in aqueous solutions of moderate to high ionic strengths. Emulsifying, dispersing and suspending are important processes in the removal of biopharmaceutical residues as many, especially some proteins and lipids, are fairly hydrophobic and tend to precipitate in aqueous cleaning solutions.

Sequestering

This process involves the solubilization of mineral salts (often with calcium, magnesium, manganese or iron as the cation) which precipitate in aqueous solutions of cleaning agents, especially those that are alkaline. These mineral salts are often polyvalent and may be soluble in pure water, but precipitate in cleaning solution due to pH, a solubility product relationship and/or elevated temperature. Sequestering agents, or chelants, can help to solubalize these mineral salts by complexing with the polyvalent cations likely to precipitate. Commonly used chelants include sodium salts of ethylene diamine tetra acetic acid (EDTA) and other specific organic acid salts. Even though chelating agents were first used for automatic cleaning because of hard water, this technology can be of use in the cleaning of biopharmaceutical equipment as well. This is true even for systems which use purified water (free from mineral salts) for cleaning because salts with polyvalent cations may be used as in-process materials, such as buffers and media components, and these may consequently require sequestering for effective removal.

Cleaning Agents and Their Functions

The practical application of the cleaning processes described above involves the selection of cleaning agents that provide the means for the residue removal mechanisms appropriate to a specific process or residue. The following is a review of cleaning agents commonly in use in the biopharmaceutical industry and the role(s) that they play in residue removal.

Alkaline Cleaners

This group of cleaning agents typically includes soda ash, sodium hydroxide, potassium hydroxide, tri-sodium phosphate and sodium metasilicate. Alkaline cleaners are often used for dissolving, saponifying and peptizing processes with varying degrees of efficacy depending upon the specific residue and alkaline cleaner.

Sodium hydroxide is often a major constituent of liquid cleaners for automatic cleaning systems as it has good dissolving, saponifying and peptizing power (especially in the presence of chlorine), and it is highly germicidal and relatively inexpensive. However, sodium hydroxide lacks sequestering, emulsifying and dispersing action, it is not free-rinsing, and it is very corrosive to many non-stainless metals.

Potassium hydroxide has many of the same properties of sodium hydroxide but it is more free-rinsing. Because of this, potassium hydroxide is also often used in alkaline cleaners for clean-in- place (CIP) applications; however, it is more expensive than sodium hydroxide.

Tri-sodium phosphate is used as a source of alkalinity in liquid cleaners for automatic cleaning systems as it can have fair to good dissolving, saponifying and peptizing power (especially in the presence of chlorine), and good sequestering, disbursing and emulsifying capabilities. Tri-sodium phosphate is expensive as compared to other sources of alkalinity and it can be corrosive to some non-stainless metals, but it is relatively free-rinsing.

Sodium metasilicate is also used as a source of alkalinity in some liquid cleaners for automatic cleaning systems as it has fair to good dissolving, saponifying and peptizing power, fair sequestering capability, and good to excellent dispersing and emulsifying capabilities. Sodium metasilicate has the unusual property of being strongly alkaline but relatively non-corrosive, protective to some soft metals, such as aluminum, brass and copper, from other strong alkalis. Sodium metasilicate is relatively expensive as compared to other sources of alkalinity and can produce precipitates of calcium and magnesium silicates if used in very hard water.

Chlorinated alkaline cleaners are often quite effective in the degradation of proteins. Chlorine levels of 50 to 200 ppm can markedly increase the peptizing ability of many alkaline cleaners. However, chlorine may not be compatible with some specific sources of alkalinity; certain mixtures may result in insoluble precipitates. Chlorine at these levels in a solution of high pH is not a bactericidal agent, nor is it corrosive to stainless steel surfaces.

It is not uncommon for more than one of the compounds discussed above to be used in combination to impart specific properties to the resulting formulated alkaline cleaner. These formulated cleaners also often contain wetting, emulsifying and suspending agents so that one liquid product can provide all of the cleaning mechanisms required for a given application.

Acidic Cleaners

This group of cleaning agents typically includes organic acids such as citric, acetic and tartaric, and inorganic acids such as phosphoric and nitric. Acidic cleaners are typically effective in dissolving (especially mineral precipitates and sugars) and peptizing (especially for some heat precipitated proteinaceous residues).

Phosphoric acid or phosphoric and nitric "blends" are often used as a neutralizing and demineralizing agent following cleaning with an alkaline detergent. This is because many alkaline detergents, even those with chelants, may cause the precipitation of polyvalent mineral salt residues that the acidic cleaners effectively remove.

Acidic cleaners are often comprised of inorganic and/or organic acids and wetting agents. To be effective in many applications, an acidic detergent should produce a pH of 2.5 or less in the final cleaning solution. Acidic cleaners are sometimes used as a washing agents prior to, or in place of alkaline detergents, especially where heat treated and/or complex proteinaceous residues are present. However, chlorine is never used with acidic detergents as it is very corrosive when present in low pH solutions and under these circumstances chlorine gas, which is toxic, can be released.

Acidic cleaners are also often used as neutralizing agents following alkaline cleaners. This is because many of the most effective alkaline cleaning agents are not free-rinsing and their complete removal would require relatively large quantities of rinsing water. Slightly acidified rinses, which may or may not be recirculated, are often used for the dual purpose of de-mineralization and neutralization. In these cases, a simple acid cleaner comprised of only pure phosphoric acid or a phosphoric and nitric "blend," without wetting agents or other cleaning agents, is often used.

Wetting Agents

These compounds are components of most detergents used for automated cleaning systems. Wetting agents, often in very small quantities, lower the surface tension of cleaning solutions very significantly, thus increasing their ability to penetrate and degrade residues. Wetting agents can also provide some emulsifying and suspending capability but these processes are often more economically accomplished by other compounds discussed below. Wetting agents for use with automated cleaning systems should be readily soluble in cold water, heat stable, effective over a wide range of pH and non-foaming. The non-foaming property of wetting agents used for automatic cleaning is of critical importance as foaming can make recirculation cleaning ineffective, and in extreme cases impossible. Three general categories of wetting agents meeting these criteria are in common use in automatic cleaning system detergents. These include anionic, non-ionic and cationic wetting agents.

Anionic wetting agents are in common use in many types of detergents. These compounds include sulfated alcohols and alkyl aryl sulfonates, of which many variations exist with specific properties for specialized applications. A common example is sodium lauryl sulfate. Anionic surfactants typically have excellent emulsification capabilities but they also tend to foam. Because of their foaming properties, anionic wetting agents have limited application for CIP cleaning.

Cationic wetting agents are also used in detergents. Well known examples are the quaternary ammonium compounds, which may also be used separately as sanitizing agents. These compounds are sometimes not as effective at wetting as some of the others discussed in this section, but they may be used due to their compatibility with other cleaning agents in a formulated detergent.

Non-ionic wetting agents, as their name suggests, have no net charge. They are often comprised of polyalcohols and they become less soluble in water with increased temperature due to the dissociation of hydrogen bonds. When a non–ionic surfactant becomes insoluble, it turns cloudy, and the temperature at which this happens is know as its cloud point. The cloud point temperature is specific to individual surfactants. At, and some what above their cloud point temperature, non–ionic surfactants are non foaming and may actually exhibit de-foaming properties. At temperatures significantly above their cloud point, non-ionic surfactants can become so insoluble that they produce an oily film and become a residue themselves. Non-ionic surfactants are used in a wide range of alkaline and acidic cleaners for CIP cleaning, and they are often complex organic compounds that are synthesized for specific detergent applications.

Emulsifying and Suspending Agents

This group of cleaning agents often includes simple phosphates, complex phosphates, metasilicates and some of the wetting agents discussed above. Their purpose is to emulsify, disperse and suspend residues removed from equipment surfaces so that they do not re-deposit. Since simple phosphates and metasilicates have other cleaning uses, they may be present in formulated detergents for other primary purposes, secondarily providing emulsifying and suspending capabilities.

Complex phosphates, including tetrasodium pyrophosphate, sodium tripolyphosphate, sodium tetraphosphate, sodium hexametaphosphate and others, have fair to excellent emulsifying and suspending properties depending upon the residue, and they can have some peptizing power. Complex phosphates also have specific sequestering activity, and when formulated properly can prevent calcium and magnesium salt deposits in alkaline cleaning solutions.

Specialty and Non-Aqueous Cleaners

While the vast majority of residues encountered in the biopharmaceutical manufacturing can be removed using one or more of the cleaning agents discussed above, others can require residue specific compounds for effective removal.

These can include enzymes, inorganic catalysts and other agents. As one can imagine, these types of cleaning compounds can be expensive and time consuming to develop and use, and should likely be used as a "last resort" if more conventional cleaning agents are ineffective.

Some residues can require the use of non–aqueous cleaners for effective removal. These include organic solvents such as methanol, ethanol, toluene, hexane and others. The use of these solvents for spray cleaning presents difficulties due to their flammability and the possibility of explosion. Where organic solvents are used, the processing equipment, cleaning equipment, utility systems, and their piping and instrumentation will have to be specially specified, designed and constructed to deal with the hazard of possible explosion, resulting in substantial additional costs. The disposal of these types of cleaners following use can also be problematic. As with the residue specific cleaners, non-aqueous systems should be avoided if possible.

AUTOMATIC CLEANING STRATEGIES

Automated cleaning systems are used widely for the cleaning of biopharmaceutical processing equipment and piping systems, with the goal being that of the reduction of post production and detergent residues to acceptable levels. As noted above, the attainment of this goal involves the design and selection of equipment and interconnecting piping such that it can be automatically cleaned, and an understanding of the physical and chemical properties of the residues and the likely cleaning processes required for their removal. Based upon this information, an appropriate cleaning strategy can be selected that will result in reliable and repeatable cleaning, efficient utility usage (including purified water, Water for Injection (WFI), and steam), minimal cleaning agent usage, and minimal cleaning time. Issues such as physical versus chemical cleaning, factors affecting cleaning efficiency, and other process and residue specific criteria should be reviewed prior to the selection of a cleaning strategy or system.

Chemical Versus Physical Cleaning

Automated cleaning systems used to clean biopharmaceutical processing equipment and piping systems often rely primarily on chemical means for residue removal from product contact surfaces, although both chemical and physical action are typically used to some extent. Chemical cleaning involves the removal of residues from equipment surfaces by cleaning agent induced erosion and typically does not rely much on physical action or external energy. Cleaning systems that employ primarily chemical means for residue removal most often use fixed-type spray devices for solution distribution. The fixed-type spray devices, when used for vessel cleaning, are often configured such that they spray only the top 20 to 30 percent of the tank. Since these spray devices operate at relatively low pressures (25 psig or less), they provide limited physical cleaning action and are primarily solution distributors that rely on the chemically induced erosion of residues from the surfaces that they cover. The cleaning of the rest of the vessel, not being directly covered by solution from the spray device, is also accomplished by chemical erosion, provided by the falling film of cleaning solution. Fixed-type spray devices can be fabricated to the same standards as the vessels such that they are completely self cleaning and self draining and thus are acceptable for product contact and permanent installation.

Chemical erosion works well for removal of many biopharmaceutical residues, even those "bonded" to equipment surfaces by heat treatment, chemical reaction and other means. However, some residue deposits are so tenacious that physical action (impingement), in addition to chemical erosion, may be required for efficient removal. In these cases, high pressure (typically greater than 50 psig) rotating spray devices may be used to apply both cleaning solutions and external energy for residue removal. However, if impingement is needed for residue removal, it will be required for all equipment surfaces. The need to directly spray all equipment surfaces may result in longer cleaning cycles. Because of the mechanism needed for rotation, rotating sprays are typically comprised of some non-sanitary components, and this necessitates their removal following cleaning. Also, it is essential to their performance that rotating spray devices turn properly during cleaning and thus motion sensors should be used with them to detect mechanical failure. These issues combined with other disadvantages inherent to rotating sprays make them less desirable than fixed-type sprays for many hygienic applications.

Factors Affecting Cleaning Efficiency

The factors affecting cleaning efficiency include cleaning solution temperature, cleaning agent concentration, cleaning solution contact time and external energy. Each of these, to an extent, has a direct relationship with cleaning efficiency and, because of their significant effects on cleaning, are often used as the means for cleaning cycle tuning.

Cleaning Solution Temperature

This factor can have a significant effect on cleaning efficiency because increased temperature increases reaction rates (such as for dissolving, saponifying and peptizing processes), decreases cleaning solution viscosity, increases the solubility of many residues, decreases the strength of the bonds between some residues and surfaces, and increases the activity of some surfactants (especially non-ionics). However, increasing the cleaning temperature only has a positive effect to a point because of protein denaturation. Cleaning temperatures above a certain point can actually decrease cleaning efficiency due to protein precipitation and deposition, and due to surfactant insolubility. This "maximum" temperature for biopharmaceutical residues is often in the range of 45° to 70°C; however, it is unique to specific residues and detergents.

Cleaning Agent Concentration

This factor also has a substantial effect on cleaning efficiency, especially in systems relying entirely on chemical erosion for residue removal. As with temperature, to an extent, increased cleaning agent concentration will increase cleaning efficiency. The goal in the tuning of this factor is to find the minimum concentration of cleaning agent(s) that will assure reliable, repeatable, efficient and economical cleaning. This is of increasing significance with regard to EPA regulations concerning pH of effluent streams and other discharge requirements. When cleaning difficulties are encountered, in addition to considering increasing the cleaning agent concentration, the types of cleaning agents used and their sequence of application should be evaluated carefully with regard to residue characteristics and likely required cleaning mechanisms. This will help to ensure that appropriate cleaning agents are chosen so that they may be used efficiently.

Typical biopharmaceutical residues may be removed with alkaline cleaner (including other agents such as surfactants, sequesterants, emulsifiers, etc.) concentrations for the detergent wash in the range of 1,500 to 7,500 ppm as sodium hydroxide, and acidic cleaner concentrations for the acidified wash in the range of 1,000 to 2,500 ppm as phosphoric acid.

Cleaning Solution Contact Time

Adequate cleaning solution contact time is essential for efficient cleaning. As with the other factors discussed above, at a given detergent concentration and solution temperature, there is a minimum amount of cleaning solution contact time required for the reliable and repeatable removal of each specific residue from equipment surfaces. Values greatly in excess of this minimum are not likely to greatly enhance residue removal and will probably be too time consuming to be economically reasonable. For biopharmaceutical residues, the detergent wash step of the cycle is often in the range of 20 to 60 minutes in length, and the acidified wash step of the cycle is often in the range of 5 to 15 minutes in length. If alkaline and acidified wash times are substantially in excess of these ranges, adjustment of one or more of the other factors affecting cleaning efficiency should be considered.

External Energy

This factor is important with regard to cleaning efficiency, especially for systems relying on impingement and chemical erosion for residue removal. For manually cleaned equipment, this factor would refer to the physical scrubbing action of brushes or other cleaning tools, but in automatic cleaning systems external energy involves turbulence, velocity and pressure on equipment surfaces and in piping systems. For some time, a minimum velocity of 5 ft/sec has been used as a guideline for cleaning piping systems, even though this does not yield a consistent Reynolds Number, a well established measurement of turbulence, with changes in pipe diameter. As a general guideline, effective piping system cleaning can be accomplished at Reynolds Numbers of 30,000 to 35,000, and at 200–300 with free falling films on equipment surfaces. For impingement cleaning, the pressure at the contact point between the cleaning solution and the equipment surface is a critical factor as solution pressure is a major means of residue removal.

Cleaning solution temperature, cleaning agent concentration, cleaning solution contact time and external energy are interrelated with respect to cleaning efficiency. The adjustment of any one of the factors will have an effect on the others, and thus they can be used very effectively in the tuning and optimization of cleaning cycles.

Choosing Appropriate Cleaning Strategies

It is essential that processing equipment, especially vessels, and piping systems are designed and installed such that they *can* be automatically cleaned. This may seem obvious but it is not uncommon to find biopharma-ceutical equipment that, because of design and/or installation problems, is not capable of being automatically cleaned. For vessels, this is often due to poorly located nozzles, difficult to clean appurtenances within the equipment, misapplied spray devices and lack of drainability. For piping systems, this is often due to excessively long dead ends, poorly designed CIP circuits, non-sanitary components and pitch problems. In either case, the cleanability of the processing system and its interconnecting piping is a critical factor in the successful application of CIP technology.

Another important factor in selecting a cleaning strategy is the nature of the residue to be removed. For example, if the residue is not bonded tightly to the equipment surfaces and readily soluble in aqueous cleaning solutions, a rudimentary cleaning cycle with fixed-type spray devices and simple cleaning agent(s) would likely be chosen. However, if the residue were not soluble in aqueous cleaning solutions and tightly bonded to equipment surfaces, a complicated cleaning cycle using impingement and/or complex cleaning agents might be required. While this is a rather simplistic example, these are the types of issues that should be addressed in the selection of an appropriate cleaning strategy.

Another important consideration is the extent to which cleaning equipment is automated. For instance, if complex cleaning sequences are required due to equipment and/or residue constraints, a relatively high degree of cleaning system automation may be needed. Clean-in-place (CIP) and clean-out-of-place (COP) systems typically run more reliably and repeatedly when they are automated. CIP system automation will result in added capital costs, but operating costs may be reduced. A reasonable guideline might be that CIP systems should be automated to the point that manual operator actions are not required for routine system functions except starting cycles.

TYPICAL CIP CLEANING PROGRAM SEQUENCES FOR VESSELS AND PIPING

Typical automatic cleaning sequences for biopharmaceutical processing equipment and interconnecting piping often include a pre-rinse, an alkaline detergent wash, a post rinse, an acidified wash and a final rinse. The following is a relatively detailed description of a typical biopharmaceutical CIP sequence, and while it is relatively specific, it is only an example as many variations of cleaning sequences are used depending upon the equipment being cleaned, the nature of the residues and other factors discussed above. The program steps for this and the other types of cycles that will be discussed are depicted in Figure 2.1.

Pre-Rinse(s) and Drain(s)

Pre-rinsing is often the first step of the sequence and typically involves the rinsing of equipment surfaces with ambient domestic or purified water. For single use solution recovery CIP systems, this liquid may be recovered wash water from the previous cycle, although this is not common due to the concerns about cross contamination. The rinsing solution is typically sent to drain following contact with the equipment surfaces and not recirculated. The purpose of this step is to remove the bulk of the residue, which is often readily soluble in water and which often comprises the majority of the total residue in the system. Pre-rinsing waters are often not heated so that they do not cause denaturation of proteinaceous residues, which can make them much more difficult to remove.

The pre-rinse may be operated continuously, which is common for cycles that only involve piping and/or equipment that is to be cleaned by flooding or pressure washing. Or, the pre-rinse may be done in segments, or bursts, with

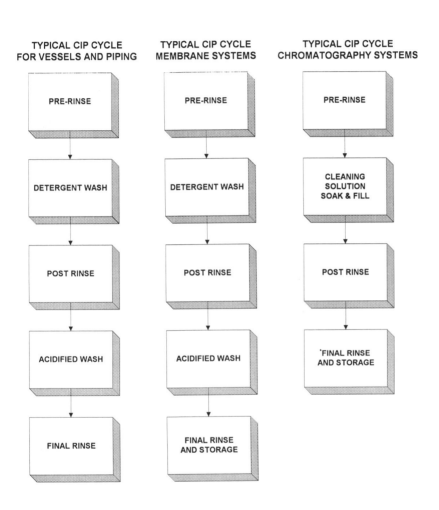

Figure 2.1
Typical Biopharmaceutical Cleaning Cycles

drain steps in between. Often this is done for cycles in which vessels are cleaned so that they may be drained completely between rinses, thus allowing residues to be more completely flushed away.

The endpoint for the pre-rinse(s) is often based upon totalized volume or elapsed time, but can be based upon on-line turbidity or conductivity or return flow, although this is rare. During an early portion of the pre-rinse, a return flow probe is often used to confirm that the cleaning circuit is properly configured prior to continuing and adding cleaning agents.

The pre-rinse drain(s) are used to allow the equipment being cleaned and the CIP return piping to be drained prior to the next step of the cycle, which may be another pre–rinse or a detergent wash. In either event, the purpose is to assure that rinsing water containing the bulk residues has completely drained from the equipment being cleaned, thus minimizing carry-over and possible re-deposition. A pre-rinse drain typically follows each pre-rinse.

The pre-rinse drain(s) are performed by stopping the "supply side" of the CIP unit and allowing its "return side" to continue to operate. The endpoint for pre-rinse drain(s) is often elapsed time, but level sensors in the equipment being cleaned and other instrumental methods may be used.

The liquids that are not recirculated in this and subsequent cycle steps may flow to a "bio-kill" system rather than to process drains if their containment is required. This does not typically require substantive changes to the operation of the system(s) but may place flow rate and quantity constraints on cleaning unit(s). Additionally as a method of containment, some equipment may require steam sterilization prior to cleaning and this can make cleaning much more difficult due to residue denaturation and other factors.

Detergent Wash and Drain

The detergent wash step of the sequence is used to remove the materials not removed by the pre-rinse(s), and this may constitute a small to moderate quantity of the total residues. The solution may or may not be recirculated depending upon the CIP system design.

For recirculating systems, the detergent wash is started by the transfer of an appropriate quantity of domestic or purified water into the CIP supply and return piping and the equipment being cleaned so that the circuit can be "closed" and recirculation initiated. For re-use systems, the liquid used for recirculation may be recycled wash water, but this is not common due to concerns about cross contamination. Once recirculation is established, detergent(s) is added and the solution is typically heated. The detergent is often an alkaline cleaner, but acidic and other cleaners may be used, with the determination being made depending upon the characteristics of the specific residues. The detergent addition setpoint may be based upon volume or conductivity.

For non-recirculating systems, the detergent wash is similar to the pre-rinse(s) in that the domestic or purified water used contacts the equipment surfaces only once and is then sent to drain. The difference is that detergent is continuously fed into the CIP supply stream, and the water may be heated. As with recirculating systems, the detergent is often an alkaline cleaner, but acidic and other cleaners may be used, again with this selection being made depending upon the characteristics of the specific residues. The detergent addition is often accomplished by a continuous feed metering pump or venturi feeder.

The endpoint for the detergent wash, for both recirculating and non-recirculating systems, is typically totalized volume or elapsed time. This endpoint along with the detergency and heating setpoints provides the ability to adjust factors affecting cleaning efficiency, including solution contact time, solution detergency and solution temperature.

The detergent wash drain is used to allow the equipment being cleaned and the CIP return piping to be drained of the residue and detergent laden solutions prior to the next step of the cycle, which is typically a post rinse. The purpose is to assure that washing solution containing the residues and detergent has completely drained from the equipment being cleaned, thus minimizing carry-over and making post rinsing more effective, especially where alkaline detergents have been used.

The drain step in the sequence is performed by stopping the "supply side" of the CIP unit and allowing its "return side" to continue to operate. Often the CIP supply piping is purged with compressed air during, or prior to, the detergent wash drain. The endpoint for the detergent wash drain is often elapsed time, but level sensors in the equipment being cleaned and other instrumental methods may be used.

Post Rinse(s) and Drains

The post rinse step of the sequence is used to rinse equipment surfaces with ambient domestic or purified water following the detergent wash. This rinsing solution is typically sent to the drain following contact with the equipment surfaces and not recirculated. The purpose of this step is to remove the residue and detergent clinging to equipment and piping surfaces following the detergent wash drain. Post rinsing waters are typically not heated.

Like the pre-rinse, the post rinse can be operated continuously, which is common for cycles where only piping and/or equipment is to be cleaned by flooding or pressure washing. Or, the post rinse may be done in segments, or bursts, with drain steps in between. This is common for cycles in which vessels are cleaned so that they may be drained completely between rinses, thus allowing detergent and residues to be more completely flushed away.

The endpoint for the post rinse(s) is often based upon totalized volume or elapsed time, but can be based upon return line turbidity, pH or conductivity, although this is rare.

The post rinse drain(s) is used to allow the equipment being cleaned and the CIP return piping to be drained prior to the next step of the cycle, which is often an acidified wash. The purpose is to assure that rinsing water containing detergent and residues has completely drained from the equipment being cleaned, thus minimizing carry-over and mixing with the acidified solution that is to follow. A post rinse drain typically follows each post rinse.

As with the other drain steps, this step in the sequence is performed by stopping the "supply side" of the CIP unit and allowing its "return side" to continue to operate. The endpoint for pre-rinse drains is often elapsed time, but level sensors in the equipment being cleaned and other instrumental methods may be used.

Acidified Wash and Drain

This step of the sequence is employed if an alkaline cleaning agent was used in the detergent wash described above. The purpose of the acidified wash is to neutralize any remaining alkalinity and to remove any mineral deposits and other residues not soluble in the alkaline detergent solution used in the detergent wash step of the sequence. The solution may or may not be recirculated depending upon the CIP system design.

For recirculating systems, the acidified wash is started by the transfer of an appropriate quantity of domestic or purified water into the CIP supply and return piping and the equipment being cleaned so that the circuit may be "closed" and recirculation can be initiated. Once recirculation is established, an acidic cleaning agent is added and the solution is typically not heated. The detergent addition setpoint may be based upon volume or conductivity. The solution may or may not be heated.

For non-recirculating systems, the acidified wash is similar to the pre-rinse(s) and post rinse(s) in that the domestic or purified water used contacts the equipment surfaces only once and is then sent to drain. The difference is that acidic cleaner is continuously fed into the CIP supply stream, and the water may or may not be heated. The detergent addition is often accomplished by a continuous feed metering pump or venturi feeder.

The endpoint for the acidified wash, for both recirculating and non-recirculating systems, is typically totalized volume or elapsed time.

The acidified wash drain is used to allow the equipment being cleaned and the CIP return piping to be drained of the acidified solution prior to the next step of the cycle, which is the final rinse. The purpose is to assure that washing solution containing the residues and acidic cleaner has been completely drained from the equipment being cleaned, thus minimizing carry-over and making final rinsing more effective.

As with the other drain steps, this step in the sequence is performed by stopping the "supply side" of the CIP unit and allowing the "return side" to continue to operate. Often the CIP supply piping is purged with compressed air during, or prior to, the acidified wash drain. The endpoint for the detergent wash drain is often elapsed time, but level sensors in the equipment being cleaned and other instrumental methods may be used.

Final Rinse(s) and Drains

This step of the sequence is used to rinse equipment surfaces with ambient domestic, purified or WFI water following the acidified wash. This rinsing solution is typically sent to the drain following contact with the equipment surfaces and not recirculated. The purpose of this step is to remove any residual acidic cleaner that may be clinging to equipment and piping surfaces following the acidified wash drain. Final rinsing waters may or may not be heated.

As with the pre-rinse(s) and post rinse(s), the final rinse(s) may be operated continuously or they may be done in segments, or bursts, with drain steps in between. This is common for cycles in which vessels are cleaned so that they may be drained completely between rinses, thus allowing acidic cleaner and other residues to be more completely flushed away.

The endpoint for the final rinse(s) is often based upon totalized volume or elapsed time, but can be based upon on-line turbidity, pH or conductivity, although this is rare.

The final rinse drain(s) is used to allow the equipment being cleaned and the CIP return piping to be drained prior to the end of the cycle. The purpose is to assure that final rinsing water has completely drained from the equipment being cleaned prior to cleaning system shut-down. A final rinse drain typically follows each final rinse.

As with the other drain steps, this step in the sequence is performed by stopping the "supply side" of the CIP unit and allowing the "return side" to continue to operate. Often the CIP supply piping is purged by air during, or prior to, the final rinse drain, thus leaving the CIP supply and return piping, and the equipment surfaces being cleaned essentially dry at the completion of the cycle. The endpoint for the final rinse drain(s) is often elapsed time, but return line resistivity, conductivity, pH and other instrumental methods are also often used.

TYPICAL CIP CLEANING PROGRAM SEQUENCES FOR MEMBRANE SYSTEMS

Typical automatic cleaning sequences for membrane systems often include a pre-rinse, an alkaline detergent wash, a post rinse, an optional acidified wash, a final rinse and final fill with storage solution. The following is a relatively detailed description of a typical CIP sequence for a biopharmaceutical processing membrane system, and while it is relatively specific, it is only an example as many variations of cleaning sequences are used depending upon the membrane being cleaned, the nature of the residues and other factors discussed above.

Pre-Rinse(s)

This is the first step of the sequence and typically involves the rinsing of the membrane surfaces with ambient purified water or a buffer solution. The rinsing water often originates from a process vessel or other dedicated tank that provides a low pressure water or solution supply to the membrane system pump(s). This configuration can help to protect the membranes from damage due to possible CIP or purified water system pressure surges. The rinsing solution from both the permeate and retentate sides is typically not recirculated. Rather, it is sent to the drain following contact with the membrane surfaces. The purpose of this step is to remove the bulk of the residue, which is often readily soluble in water and which can comprise a majority of the total residue in the system. Pre-rinsing waters are not often heated so that they do not cause denaturation of proteinaceous residues, which can make them much more difficult to remove.

The rinsing water may flow in the direction of the process flow, in reverse, or a combination of the two depending upon the membrane system design. The pre-rinse is typically operated continuously until most readily soluble residues are flushed away. The endpoint for the pre-rinse(s) is often based upon totalized volume or elapsed time, but can be based upon on-line turbidity, conductivity, UV or other instrumental methods.

Detergent Wash

This step of the sequence is used to remove the materials not removed by the pre-rinse(s), and this often may constitute a small to moderate quantity of the total residues. The solution may or may not be recirculated depending upon the membrane system design.

The washing solution is often batched in the specific process vessel or dedicated tank mentioned above, and is typically comprised of purified or WFI water with added cleaning agent(s). These cleaning agents may be alkaline, but often pure sodium hydroxide or potassium hydroxide is used rather than formulated detergents, because surfactants, chlorine and other cleaning agents may be harmful to the membranes. The washing solution is typically recirculated and heated, although single pass cleaning of membrane systems is not uncommon, and some membrane materials have strict temperature specifications requiring un-heated washing solutions.

The endpoint for the detergent wash is typically totalized volume or elapsed time. As with the cleaning of processing vessels and piping, this endpoint along with the detergency and heating setpoints provide the ability to adjust factors affecting cleaning efficiency, including solution contact time, solution detergency and solution temperature, and thus these parameters should be easily changeable and protected on a per cycle basis.

Post Rinse(s)

This step of the sequence is used to rinse the membrane surfaces with ambient purified or WFI water. As with the pre-rinse(s), the rinsing water often originates from a process vessel or other dedicated tank that provides a low pressure water or solution supply to the membrane system pump(s). This rinsing solution from both the permeate and retentate sides is typically sent to the drain following contact with the membrane surfaces and not recirculated. The purpose of this step is to remove the cleaning agent(s) and in-process material residues following the detergent wash step. Post rinsing waters are often not heated.

As with the pre-rinse(s), the rinsing water may flow in the direction of the process flow, or in reverse, or a combination of the two depending upon the membrane system design. The post rinse is typically operated continuously until the detergent and in-process residues are flushed away. The endpoint for the pre-rinse(s) is often based upon totalized volume or elapsed time, but can be based upon on-line turbidity, conductivity, UV or other instrumental methods.

Acidified Wash

This optional step of the sequence is used to neutralize residual alkalinity and remove mineral deposits that may have formed during the detergent wash. The solution may or may not be recirculated depending upon the membrane system design.

The acidified wash solution, if used, is often batched in the specific process vessel or dedicated tank mentioned above, and is typically composed of purified or WFI water with added cleaning agent(s). These cleaning agents are typically pure, weak acids such as phosphoric or acetic, rather than formulated acidic cleaners because surfactants and other cleaning agents can be harmful to the membranes. The acidified washing solution is typically recirculated and not heated, although single pass cleaning of membrane systems is not uncommon, and some membranes may require heated acidic washes for effective cleaning. The endpoint for the acidified wash is typically totalized volume or elapsed time.

Final Rinse(s)

This step of the sequence is used to rinse the membrane surfaces with ambient purified or WFI water. As with the pre-rinses(s) and post rinse(s), the rinsing water often originates from a process vessel or other dedicated tank. This rinsing solution from both the permeate and retentate sides is typically sent to the drain following contact with the membrane surfaces and not recirculated. The purpose of this step is to remove residual acidified cleaning agent and/or in-process material residues following the acidified wash step. Final rinsing waters are not often heated.

As with the pre-rinse(s) and post rinse(s), the rinsing water may flow in the direction of the process flow, or in reverse, or a combination of the two depending upon the membrane system design. The final rinse is typically operated continuously until the acidic cleaner and in-process residues are flushed away. The endpoint for the pre-rinse(s) is often based upon totalized volume or elapsed time, but can be based upon on-line turbidity, conductivity, UV or other instrumental methods.

Final Storage

This step of the sequence is used to completely immerse all membrane surfaces in a storage solution that protects them from degradation and is bactericidal.

The storage solution is often batched in the specific process vessel or dedicated tank mentioned above, and is typically composed of purified or WFI water with added storage agent(s). Pure sodium hydroxide or potassium hydroxide are often used as many membrane materials are alkaline stable, and the strong bases provide the bacteriostatic capabilities required. Concentrations ranging from 0.2 to 1.0 N are not uncommon. This storage method provides a very safe way of protecting membrane systems; however, it does mandate that they are cleaned both prior to and following contact with in-process materials.

TYPICAL CIP CLEANING PROGRAM SEQUENCES FOR CHROMATOGRAPHY SYSTEMS

Typical automatic cleaning sequences for chromatography systems often include a pre-rinse, an alkaline fill and soak, a post rinse, and final fill with storage solution. The following is a relatively detailed description of a typical CIP sequence for a biopharmaceutical processing chromatography system, and while it is relatively specific, it is only an example as many variations of cleaning sequences are used depending upon the resin and column being cleaned, the nature of the residues and other factors discussed above.

Pre-Rinse(s)

This is the first step of the sequence and typically involves the rinsing of the column and resin surfaces with ambient purified water or a buffer solution. The rinsing buffer often originates from a process vessel or other dedicated tank that provides a low pressure water or buffer solution supply to the chromatography system pump(s). This rinsing solution is typically sent to the drain following contact with the resin and column surfaces and is not recirculated. The purpose of this step is to remove the bulk of the residue, which is often readily soluble in the rinsing solution. Pre-rinsing solutions are often not heated so that they do not cause denaturation of proteinaceous residues or resin degradation, and because many of these systems operate at refrigerated temperatures.

The endpoint for the pre-rinse(s) is often based upon totalized volume or elapsed time, but can be based upon on-line pH, conductivity, UV or other instrumental methods.

Cleaning Solution Fill And Soak

This step of the sequence is used to remove the residues not removed by the pre-rinse(s) The chromatography system is typically filled with cleaning solution and it is allowed to soak to provide adequate contact time for soil removal. As with membrane cleaning, the cleaning agent is often pure sodium or potassium hydroxide, because other cleaning agents such as chlorine and surfactants may foul the resin. Acidic cleaners, typically of pure weak acids, may also be used. The endpoint for the cleaning solution soak step is typically elapsed time.

Post Rinse(s)

This step of the sequence is used to rinse the resin and column surfaces with ambient or cold buffer solution, purified or WFI water. As with the pre-rinse(s), the rinsing buffer often originates from a process vessel or other dedicated tank that provides a low pressure water or buffer solution supply to the chromatography system pump(s). This rinsing solution is typically sent to the drain following contact with the resin and column surfaces and is not recirculated. The purpose of this step is to remove the cleaning solution and in-process material residues, which have been released from the resin and column surfaces during the prior cleaning cycle step. The endpoint for the post rinse(s) is often based on-line pH, conductivity, UV and/or other instrumental methods, but can also be based upon elapsed time or totalized volume.

Final Storage

This step of the sequence is used to completely immerse all resin and column surfaces in a storage solution that protects them from degradation and microbial contamination.

The storage solution is typically comprised of purified or WFI water with added storage agent(s). Pure sodium hydroxide or potassium hydroxide are often used as many resins are alkaline stable, and the strong bases provide the bacteriostatic capabilities required. Concentrations of 0.1 to 1.0 N are not uncommon. This storage method provides a very safe way of protecting chromatography systems; however, it does mandate that they are rinsed or cleaned both prior to and following contact with in-process materials.

MANUAL CLEANING

While CIP is often the method of choice for the cleaning of biopharmaceutical processing equipment, some degree of manual cleaning is nearly always required to deal with items that cannot be effectively automatically cleaned. Because of this, some attention must be given to manual cleaning and its validation and/or qualification.

Typical Manual Cleaning Methods

Manual cleaning is often accomplished by scrubbing and scouring of surfaces with brushes and other cleaning tools. Often, relatively mild detergents and low cleaning solution temperatures are used to minimize potential injury to operating personnel, and this is supplemented by the external energy supplied by the cleaning tools. The cleaning agents used for manual cleaning are often of relatively neutral pH and thus typically do not require neutralizing rinses. Manual cleaning is also accomplished by soaking, sonication, parts washers of various configurations and other methods.

Manual Cleaning Validation

Manual cleaning is generally considered to be less repeatable and reliable than automatic cleaning, and thus more difficult to validate. While many of the same validation strategies may be applied, manual cleaning relies on an operator doing the work in the same manner each time, and this is nearly impossible to monitor and control. Good documentation in the form of SOPs and training materials is essential for good results. But even with good documentation and training in place, small variations in cleaning procedures between operators may make reliability and repeatability very difficult to attain. For aseptic or sterile processes, re-assembly of parts following cleaning may present difficulties due to re-contamination.

However, even with all of the difficulties noted above, manual cleaning procedures are required for nearly every biopharmaceutical process and their validation is also required. As with automatically cleaned equipment, one should demonstrate that the cleaning method removes the in-process and cleaning agent residues that are likely to be found on the equipment surfaces, and that the cleaning procedure, when performed correctly, is reliable and repeatable. Since there are no automatic controls or instruments to monitor, good cleaning procedure documentation and training are essential to successful manual cleaning.

SUMMARY

The cleaning of biopharmaceutical processes requires a good understanding of the design and configuration of processing equipment and interconnecting piping such that it can be effectively cleaned, an understanding of the chemical and physical properties of the residues to be removed, an understanding of the processes involved in cleaning and the cleaning agents that facilitate these mechanisms, and a clear comprehension of factors affecting cleaning efficiency and their application to specific systems and cycles. All of these factors, when appropriately employed, can result in a cleaning program that is reliable, repeatable, economical and efficacious.

3

Automatic Cleaning Equipment

Automatic and semi-automatic cleaning equipment and systems are widely applied in the biopharmaceutical industry. These systems often include combinations of tanks, pumps, valves and instrumentation with varying degrees of automatic controls. The text in this section describes commonly used systems and components in terms of their overall configuration and operation, and their relative advantages and disadvantages as applied to biopharmaceutical processes.

TYPICAL CLEAN-IN-PLACE SYSTEMS

For purposes of this discussion, clean-in-place (CIP) is defined as the automatic cleaning of processing equipment, vessels, piping and in-line devices with minimal manual set-up and shut-down, and little or no operator intervention during cleaning. CIP cleaning is also characterized by the spray cleaning of vessels and pressure washing of piping and in-line devices, with the majority of soil removal being accomplished by chemical action rather than physical energy.

Portable CIP Systems

Portable CIP Systems have been applied to hygienic processes for many years. They may consist of as little as a cleaning agent feed system, water supply valves and a simple controller (see Figure 3.1), all mounted on a cart so

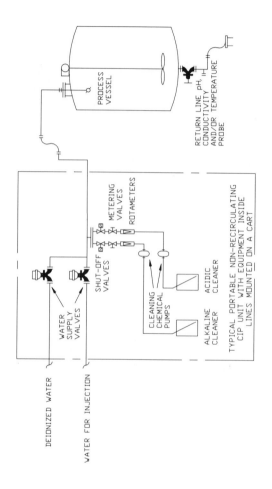

Figure 3.1
Typical Portable Non-Recirculating CIP Unit and Process Vessel

that the system can be moved to and from the process equipment and piping to be cleaned. Other Portable Systems may include the components noted above plus a recirculation tank and pump (see Figure 3.2).

Because they are designed to be moved, Portable CIP Systems require utility connections at each use point, and these utilities typically include potable and/or purified water, electrical power and steam or hot water. Also, the CIP supply and return (if required) connections typically involve flexible hoses as permanently installed piping is difficult to utilize with portable equipment.

The sprays used with Portable CIP Systems are often removable units that can be either fixed-type or rotating devices. These require installation prior to, and removal following CIP. By contrast, fixed-type spray devices, which are not typically used with Portable CIP Systems, need not be removed following cleaning.

Many Portable CIP Systems are not designed to recirculate cleaning solutions, and therefore use water, heat and cleaning agent(s) on a "once-through" basis. While this is often uneconomical, it also requires variable flow rate proportioning cleaning agent feed equipment and a relatively high capacity solution heating capability or hot water feed. In either case repeatable cleaning temperature and cleaning agent concentration may be problematic. The motive force of solution supply for these types of systems is typically the pressure of the feed water and thus the feed water pressure must be in excess of the spray device's requirements. In the case of rotating sprays, this is often greater than 65 psig, which may be difficult to attain and require additional pumping capacity, especially for WFI and USPW water systems.

Portable CIP Systems typically require a relatively low degree of control system sophistication as compared with other CIP systems. This is because most Portable CIP Systems have small numbers of devices to be controlled, such as pumps, valves and instruments, and they generally employ a very simple cleaning cycle and operating logic.

The validation of Portable CIP Systems can be both easy and difficult. For instance, since the systems typically use limited numbers of valves, pumps and instruments, and their cycles can be very simple, the Installation Qualification (IQ) and Operational Qualification (OQ) can be relatively easy and straightforward. However, since much manual set-up is typically required prior to staring a CIP cycle there is a greater opportunity for human error, thus requiring the structuring of the PQ and SOPs such that the most common pitfalls are detected and corrected, such as improper CIP supply/return connections, spray device installation errors and utility drop connection mistakes, to name a few. Portable CIP Systems are in use in the biopharmaceutical industry, especially in small scale and pilot facilities.

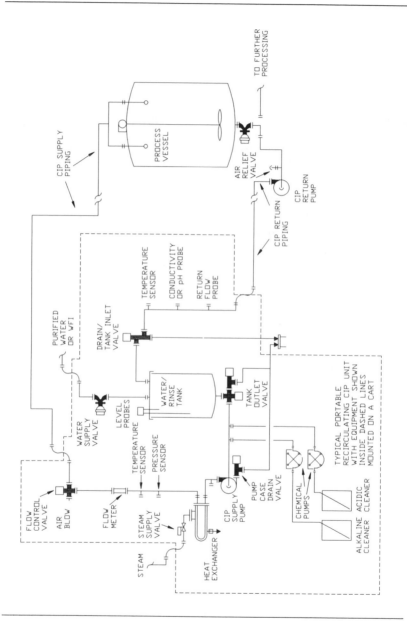

Figure 3.2
Typical Portable Recirculating CIP System with Process Vessel

Multiple-Tank Re-Use CIP Systems

As implied by their name, Multiple-Tank Re-Use CIP systems typically consist of several vessels, one for each type of cleaning solution used including each kind of water, and they are designed to re-use wash water from one cleaning cycle to the next. Their components typically include (see Figure 3.3) a supply pump, utility supply and cleaning solution distribution valves, instrumentation for recording and control, a cleaning agent feed system, and a control system. These CIP systems are often permanently installed, with permanently installed CIP supply/return and utility piping. The spray devices used with Multiple-Tank Re-Use CIP systems are typically fixed-type and are often permanently installed, although rotating sprays may be used with these systems.

Most Multiple-Tank Re-Use CIP Systems are designed to recirculate cleaning solutions, and they are also configured to re-use wash solutions from one cycle to the next. While the intent of solution re-use is to enhance the economical operation of the system, solution re-use is typically not employed in the cleaning of biopharmaceutical equipment due to concerns about residue carry-over. The ability to re-use cleaning solutions requires that the CIP system solution tank(s) have the capacity of the volume of the largest circuit in the facility. These solution vessels are often 950 to 2,000 liters (or larger) in capacity, and if re-use is not employed, the solution tank(s) capacity represents the amount of cleaning solution dumped after each cycle. Thus, Multiple-Tank Re-Use CIP Systems used in "single-use mode" consume relatively large quantities of water and cleaning agents, as compared to other types of recirculating CIP units.

In addition to the components described above, Multiple-Tank Re-Use CIP Systems can have either pumped or eductor generated return flow. The eductor-generated return flow systems have the advantage of not requiring return pumps, but an additional pump and tank is required adjacent to the other CIP tanks, pumps and valves. Since sanitary only eductors produce 17–20" of vacuum at normal operating temperatures, the CIP return lines for these systems must be relatively large, or the equipment being cleaned must be close to the CIP system, or both. By contrast, systems with pumped returns can have smaller return lines, but return pumps are required adjacent to the equipment being cleaned, and it can be difficult to get return pumps to operate properly due to air incorporation. To address this problem, low speed (1,750 rpm) centrifugal pumps with air relief valves are commonly used in the CIP return piping system. Both types of return systems are in use in the biopharmaceutical industry.

Multiple-Tank Re-Use CIP Systems typically require a moderate degree of control system sophistication as compared with other CIP systems. This is because most of these types of systems have a moderate number of devices to

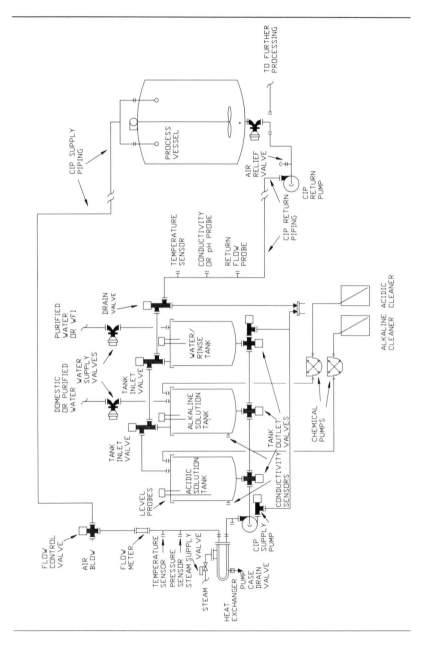

Figure 3.3
Typical Multi-Tank, Re-Use CIP System with Process Vessel

be controlled, such as pumps, valves and instruments, and they generally employ a moderately simple cleaning cycle sequence and operating logic.

The validation of Multiple-Tank Re-Use CIP Systems can be relatively easy to moderately difficult depending upon the numbers of valves, pumps and instruments used, and the complexity of their cycles. The IQ and OQ can be relatively easy and straight forward, and the PQ's difficulty is dependant upon the complexity of the cycle sequence, and the degree to which permanently installed CIP supply/return piping, utility drops and spray devices are used. While Multiple-Tank Re-Use CIP Systems are in wide use in the biopharmaceutical industry, they are not often the best choice for economical operation because their wash solution re-use feature typically cannot be used due to the potential for residue carryover between CIP circuits.

Single and Multiple-Tank Single-Use CIP Systems

Single-Tank Single-Use CIP systems typically consist of a tank used for both rinse water supply and recirculation, and they are designed to use the wash water from each cleaning cycle only once. Their components typically include (see Figure 3.4) a supply pump, utility supply and cleaning solution distribution valves, instrumentation for recording and control, a cleaning agent feed system, and a control system. These CIP systems are typically permanently installed, with permanently installed CIP supply/return and utility piping. The spray devices used with Single-Tank Single-Use CIP systems are often fixed-type and are commonly permanently installed, although rotating sprays may be used with these systems.

Most Single-Tank Single-Use CIP Systems are designed to recirculate cleaning solutions, and they are also configured to use wash solutions only once. The single-use of washing solution is often employed in the cleaning of biopharmaceutical equipment due to concerns about residue carry-over between CIP circuits. Because Single-Tank Single-Use CIP Systems formulate cleaning solutions on a per cycle basis by filling the cleaning circuit with water prior to recirculation, the capacity of a typical water supply/recirculation tank is 150 to 380 liters, or the minimum volume required to provide adequate net positive suction head to the CIP supply pump. This can result in substantial water and cleaning agent savings as compared to the Multiple-Tank Re-Use System operated in single-use mode. The formulation of cleaning solutions on a per cycle basis allows for the "tailoring" of cleaning cycle parameters to each individual circuit. This is of special significance to the removal of residues from biopharmaceutical equipment as they can vary significantly in composition and thus need significantly different cleaning cycles.

In addition to the components described above, Single-Tank Single-Use CIP Systems commonly have pumped return flow, but as with the Multiple tank Re-Use CIP Systems, it can be difficult to operate return pumps properly

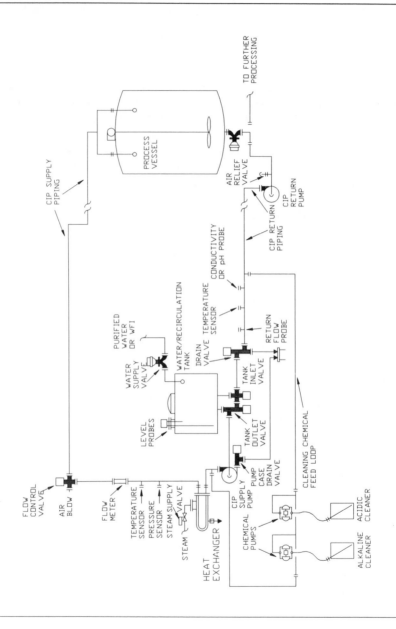

Figure 3.4
Typical Single-Tank, Single-Use CIP System with Process Vessel

due to air incorporation. To address this problem, these systems often use low speed (1,750 rpm) centrifugal pumps with air relief valves are commonly used in the CIP return piping.

Due to concerns over using a common tank for water supply and recirculation, Single-Use systems may also be configured with additional tanks for water supply and/or solution recovery (see Figure 3.5), where purified water is stored, or "spent" wash water is recovered for use as a pre-rinse for the following cycle. The solution recovery feature, however, is often not employed due to concerns about residual carry-over.

Single-Use CIP Systems typically require a moderate to high degree of control system sophistication as compared with other CIP systems. This is because most of these types of systems have a moderate number of devices to be controlled, such as pumps, valves and instruments, and they generally employ a moderately complex cleaning cycle sequence and operating logic.

As with the Multiple-Tank Re-Use CIP systems, the validation of Single-Use CIP Systems can be relatively easy to moderately difficult depending upon the numbers of valves, pumps and instruments used, and the complexity of their cycles. The IQ and OQ can be relatively easy and straight forward, and the PQ's difficulty is dependant upon the complexity of the cycle sequence, and the degree to which permanently installed CIP supply/return piping, utility drops and spray devices are used. Single-Use CIP Systems are in wide use in the biopharmaceutical industry because of their ability to provide a high degree of cycle flexibility and economical operation (see Table 3.1).

Single-Use Eductor Assisted CIP Systems

As with the Single-Use CIP systems discussed above, Single-Use Eductor Assisted CIP Systems use cleaning solutions only once. They typically consist of a single, low volume recirculation tank and one or more water supply tanks, for domestic water, WFI, or USPW. They also typically include (see Figure 3.6) a supply pump, a motive pump (for eductor operation), utility supply and cleaning solution distribution valves, instrumentation for recording and control, a cleaning agent feed system, and a control system. These CIP systems are nearly always permanently installed, with permanently installed CIP supply/return and utility piping. The spray devices used with Single-Use Eductor Assisted CIP Systems are nearly always fixed-type and are commonly permanently installed.

Single-Use Eductor Assisted CIP Systems are designed to recirculate cleaning solutions, and they are also configured to use wash solutions only once. As stated above, the single-use of washing solution is often employed in the cleaning of biopharmaceutical equipment due to concerns about residue carry-over. Because of the design of the Single-Use Eductor Assisted CIP System recirculation tank, its capacity is typically 60–75 liters, or the minimum volume

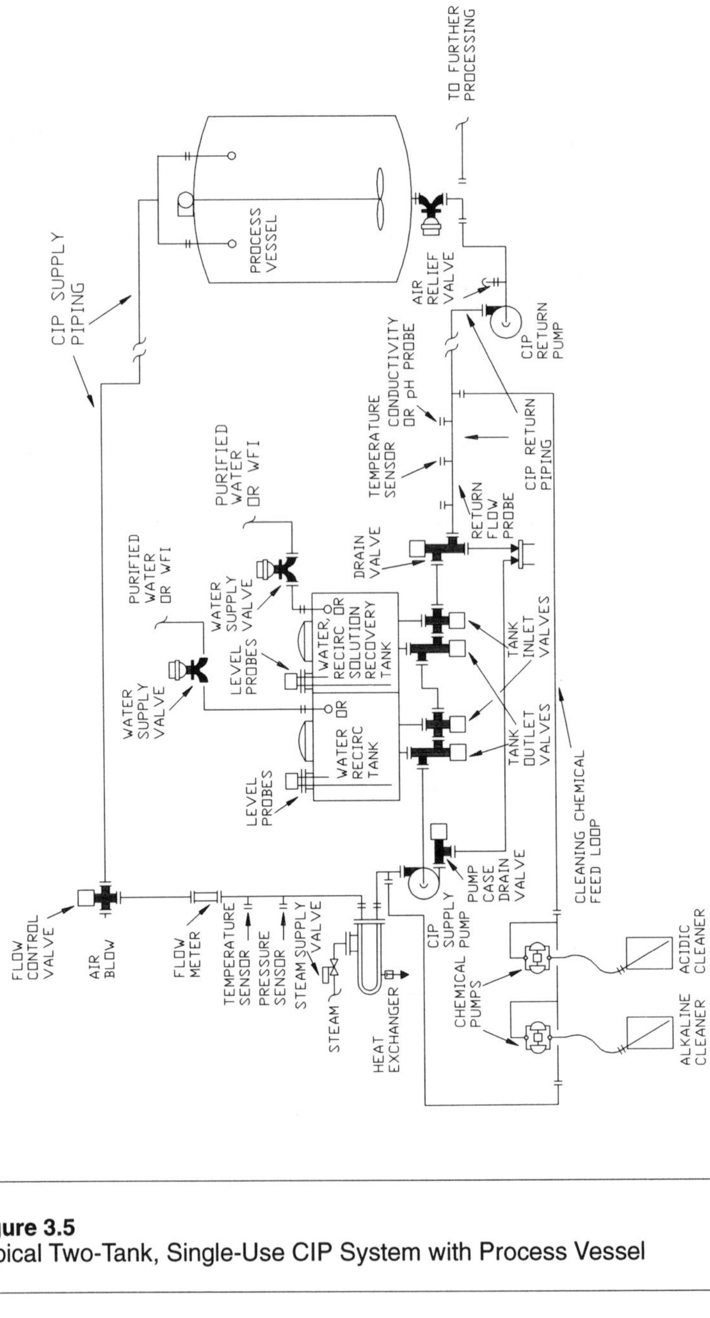

Figure 3.5
Typical Two-Tank, Single-Use CIP System with Process Vessel

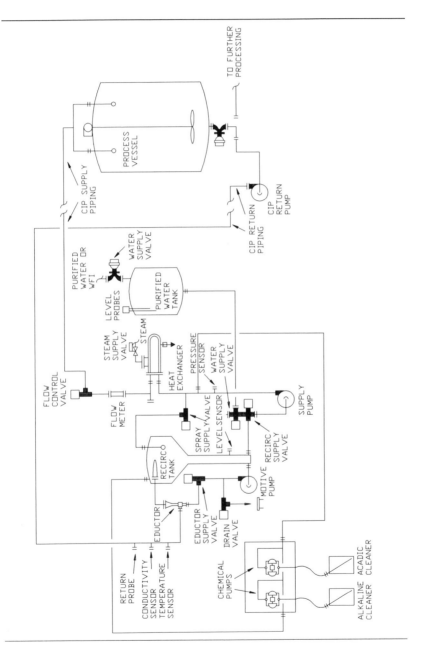

Figure 3.6
Typical Single-Use, Eductor Assisted CIP Unit

Table 3.1
CIP Systems Comparison

System Type	Control System Complexity	IQ/OQ Complexity	PQ Complexity	Biopharmaceutical Applicability
Portable Systems (Non-Recirc.)	Simple	Simple/ Moderate	Simple/ Moderate	Limited
Re-Use Systems (Recirc.)	Moderate	Moderate	Moderate/ Complex	Somewhat Limited
Single-Use Systems (Recirc.)	Moderate/ Complex	Moderate/ Complex	Moderate/ Complex	Applicable/ Very Applicable
Eductor Assisted Single-Use Systems (Recirc.)	Complex	Complex	Complex	Applicable/ Very Applicable

required to provide adequate net positive suction head to the CIP supply and motive pumps. This can result in substantial water and cleaning agent savings as compared with the other CIP systems discussed above. As with other single-use systems, the formulation of cleaning solutions on a per cycle basis allows for the "tailoring" of cleaning cycle parameters to each individual circuit. As noted above, this is of special significance to the removal of residues from biopharmaceutical equipment as they can vary significantly in composition and thus need significantly different cleaning cycles.

In addition to the components described above, Single-Use Eductor Assisted CIP Systems have pumped return flow assisted by an eductor. Because the eductor provides a vacuum on the CIP return system, it functions as a continuous pump priming device and allows for the use of high speed (3,500 rpm) pumps without air relief valves for CIP solution return. Eductor assisted systems can improve the efficacy of biopharmaceutical equipment cleaning due to their ability to produce consistent return flow from non-traditional equipment and piping configurations.

To address the concern of residue carry-over, Single-Use Eductor Assisted CIP Systems, like several of the systems discussed above, have dedicated tanks for recirculation and rinsing water supply. Solution recovery can be used with these systems, but it is not typical due to the reasons previously noted.

Single-Use Eductor Assisted CIP Systems typically require a high degree of control system sophistication as compared with other CIP systems. This is because most of these types of systems have a moderate to high number of devices to be controlled, such as pumps, valves and instruments, and they generally employ a relatively complex cleaning cycle sequence and operating logic.

The validation of Single-Use Eductor Assisted CIP Systems can be moderate to difficult. In general, these systems have higher numbers of devices to control, greater analog control requirements and more complex operating sequences. Each of these affects the IQ, OQ, and PQ in making them more complex. While relatively new as compared with other CIP systems, Single-Use Eductor Assisted CIP Systems are becoming more widely used in the biopharmaceutical industry.

TYPICAL CIP SYSTEM INSTRUMENTATION

Automated cleaning systems require instrumentation for the measurement and control of critical cleaning process variables such as solution temperature, solution flow rate, solution supply pressure, solution conductivity, CIP unit vessel liquid levels and return flow verification. Each of these system parameters is essential in controlling the primary factors of cleaning efficacy, which are solution temperature, detergency, contact time, and external energy (measured as pressure and flow rate). Thus the measurement and control of these critical cleaning process variables is essential for the repeatable and reliable operation and validation of automated cleaning equipment. The following is a brief description of typical CIP system instruments and their functions.

Temperature Sensors

Cleaning solution temperature is an important factor in the efficacy of cleaning, and thus most automated cleaning systems have instrumentation for the measurement and control of cleaning solution temperature. For cleaning systems that recirculate washing solutions, two temperature sensors are often used. One is for the control of the solution supply temperature and the other for the monitoring and recording of the return temperature. Non-recirculating systems may only use a single temperature sensor for both control and recording as they may not have a solution return flow stream to measure.

As noted above, cleaning solution temperature is a critical factor in the efficacy of cleaning and it is therefore often used as a primary indicator of cleaning cycle performance. This is especially true for the cleaning of biopharmaceutical processing equipment as the rate of removal and solubility of the residues can often be temperature dependent. The solution return temperature is considered to be the most rigorous measure of system performance as it must be at or below the temperature of the coldest spot in the cleaning circuit. It is not uncommon for the record of cleaning solution temperature to become a part of the overall records for a given production run or batch.

Sanitarily designed Resistance Temperature Detectors (RTD) are the most common devices used to measure cleaning solution temperatures. These may either be directly clamped into the cleaning piping system or they can be installed in sanitary thermal wells the are welded into the cleaning piping system. Sanitarily designed RTDs are readily available in several electronic configurations which permit their interfacing with control systems and chart recorders.

Conductivity Sensors

Cleaning solution detergency is another important factor in the efficacy of cleaning, and thus most automated cleaning systems have instrumentation for measurement of cleaning agent concentration. Since many cleaning agents are strong bases or acids, their concentration can be determined by measurement of cleaning solution conductivity. For cleaning systems that do not recirculate washing solutions, a conductivity sensor may be used for the control of the rate of cleaning agent addition. Multiple-Tank Re-Use systems that do recirculate cleaning solutions also often use a conductivity sensor to control cleaning agent addition. For many systems that do recirculate washing solutions, positive displacement pumps are used to meter exact amounts of cleaning agents into the cleaning solution, and in these cases, the conductivity sensor is required for measurement and verification (not control) of cleaning agent addition. On-line conductivity has also been used as a measure of final rinsing efficacy, but this method can lack sensitivity.

Because of its importance in cleaning efficacy, solution conductivity is often used as a primary indicator of cleaning cycle performance. Cleaning solution conductivity is often measured in the supply or return piping of the cleaning system, or it may be measured in the cleaning system solution tank(s). For cleaning systems that recirculate washing solutions, the location of the conductivity sensor is often not critical because once the solution is recirculating and mixed its cleaning agent concentration is uniform. For non-recirculating cleaning systems, the conductivity sensor must be located in the supply piping.

Sanitarily designed conductivity sensors are typically directly clamped into the cleaning piping system. They are readily available in several electronic configurations which permit their interfacing with control systems and chart recorders, and several are completely enclosed and electrodeless.

pH Sensors

Another measure of cleaning solution detergency is pH. However, because of its inherent non-linearity, pH cannot be directly correlated to cleaning agent concentration and is thus often not as useful as conductivity for measuring solution detergency. On-line pH is sometimes used as a measure of final rinsing efficacy, especially with non-recirculating systems. In these cases, the pH sensor is located at the discharge of the equipment being cleaned.

Sanitarily designed pH sensors can be directly clamped into the cleaning piping system, and they are available in several electronic configurations which permit their interfacing with control systems and chart recorders. However, on-line pH probes often require a substantial amount of maintenance, especially in CIP applications where wide variations in temperature and pH are common, and their reliability can be problematic.

CIP Supply Flow Sensors

Cleaning solution supply flow rate and totalization are important factors in the efficacy of cleaning as they are directly related to solution contact time. Thus, most automated cleaning systems have instrumentation for the measurement and control of cleaning solution supply flow rate and totalization.

Because of its importance in cleaning efficacy with respect to solution contact time, cleaning solution flow rate and totalization are often used for control and as a primary indicator of cleaning cycle performance. Cleaning solution flow rate and totalization are nearly always measured in the supply piping of the cleaning system. For purposes of flow rate control, it is common for the cleaning solution supply flow sensor to be used in conjunction with a throttling valve or variable speed pump drive. CIP flow control is typically of importance for the cleaning of biopharmaceutical processes as the scale of equipment in various areas of the same facility may vary greatly and thus require substantial variations in the cleaning solution flow rates. While not as commonly applied, the recording of solution flow rate is sometimes used as another indicator for verification of cleaning cycle performance.

Sanitarily designed flow sensors are typically directly clamped into the cleaning piping system. They are readily available in several electronic configurations which permit their interfacing with control systems and chart recorders. Several types of sensors are commonly used to measure cleaning solution flow including vortex-shedding flow meters, turbine flow meters and mass flow meters. Magnetic flow meters are not often used in biopharmaceutical CIP applications because of their inability to sense non-conductive fluids such as DI and WFI water.

CIP Supply Pressure Sensors

Cleaning solution supply pressure is an important factor in cleaning efficacy as it can be used as an indicator of system performance, typically with regard to spray device performance and solution contact time. Because of this, many automated cleaning systems have a supply line pressure sensor.

For systems that recirculate washing solutions, this pressure sensor output is also often used as an interlock by the cleaning unit's control system for heating and cleaning agent addition. The recording of cleaning solution supply pressure is often used as an indicator for verification of cleaning cycle performance, but the cleaning solution supply pressure is not often directly controlled.

Sanitarily designed pressure sensors are typically directly clamped into the cleaning piping system. They are readily available in several electronic configurations which permit their interfacing with control systems and chart recorders, with diaphragm-type pressure sensors being commonly used.

CIP Vessel Level Sensors

While not a direct indicator or control point for cleaning efficacy, the measurement and control of CIP vessel levels is very important as they directly effect the performance of the cleaning system. Nearly all automated cleaning systems include level controls for system vessels including recirculation, rinsing, water surge, and cleaning agent storage tanks. These measurements can be either digital or analog depending upon the application.

While the control of cleaning system vessel levels is often done, and these levels are often used in overall system control they are not often recorded as they would not be a meaningful indicator for verification of cleaning cycle performance.

Sanitarily designed level sensors are typically directly clamped into the cleaning system vessels, either through the top head or sidewall. They are readily available in several electronic configurations which permit their interfacing with control systems. Several types of sensors are commonly used to measure cleaning system vessel levels including digital and analog probes, differential pressure diaphragm-type sensors, bubblers, and digital and analog ultrasonic sensors.

Return Flow Switch

Because cleaning circuits typically involve "make-break" connections between the process and cleaning piping, it is possible to mis-connect cleaning supply and return piping, resulting in an incomplete circuit. The consequence of such an error could be disastrous, especially in biopharmaceutical facilities where products are typically of high value, as cleaning agents might mistakenly be mixed with product. Thus most automatic cleaning systems that recirculate washing solutions have a return flow switch to verify that a circuit exists prior to recirculation and cleaning agent addition. The return flow switch is often a conductance–based probe, installed in a self draining portion of the cleaning return piping, that senses the presence of liquid, hence return flow. This instrument output is often used as an interlock for cleaning program advance past the first pre-rinse.

TYPICAL CIP SPRAY DEVICES

Automated cleaning systems use spray devices to distribute cleaning solutions onto the interior surfaces of processing equipment which cannot be reasonably pressure washed or flooded. Spray devices may also be used to provide a means of physical soil removal by impingement. Fixed-type and rotating spray devices are used in the biopharmaceutical industry and they each have strengths and weaknesses. The following is a brief discussion of each type of device and its relative merits.

Fixed–Type Spray Devices

Fixed-type sprays most commonly used in the biopharmaceutical industry are typically comprised of hollow, spherically, or hemispherically shaped devices with small diameter holes that allow cleaning solution, under pressure, to pass through them. This configuration allows for cleaning solution to flow through the spray device via cleaning supply piping, and for the cleaning solution to be distributed through the device's small diameter holes onto the equipment surfaces being cleaned.

Because they use small diameter holes for cleaning solution distribution, fixed-type spray devices are often directionally drilled. This allows them to be fabricated such that reasonably precise quantities of cleaning solutions are supplied to specific areas of the equipment being cleaned, thus providing efficient coverage. Due to their design, fixed-type spray devices spray all of the vessel and equipment surfaces all of the time, hence resulting in continuous cleaning solution contact.

Fixed-type spray devices are typically fabricated completely of stainless steel and their surface finish (e.g., electropolished, 320 grit, < 25 Ra, etc.) and construction constraints (e.g., minimum radius corners, drainablility, self cleanability, etc.) can be to the same specifications as the vessels and equipment in which they are installed. This allows fixed-type spray devices to be permanently installed in product contacting areas.

The cleaning solution flow rate required to clean vessels using fixed-type spray devices is typically in the range of 2.0 to 2.5 gpm per circumferential foot of tank diameter. For other equipment surfaces, flow rates of 0.2 to 0.3 gpm per square foot have been reported. Since fixed-type spray devices are designed to clean surfaces by chemical rather than physical (impingement) means, they typically require supply pressures of less than 25 psig, which are relatively low, and they are typically very reliable because they have no moving parts and their spray patterns are not adversely affected by small to moderate variations in supply pressure. These characteristics make fixed-type spray device patterns relatively easy to validate.

Because fixed-type spray devices rely nearly entirely on residue removal by chemical erosion, very tenacious residues may not easily be removed because they require a moderate to high degree of impingement. However, this is not typically a problem for biopharmaceutical equipment cleaning.

Rotating Spray Devices

While not unknown in the biopharmaceutical industry, rotating spray devices are not as commonly applied as fixed-type sprays. Rotating spray devices are typically comprised of a rotating industrial-type spray device on a rotating shaft. This design allows for distribution of cleaning solution onto the equipment surfaces being cleaned with a moderate to high degree of physical cleaning (impingement) capability depending upon the supply pressure.

Because they often rotate completely (360 degrees) in one or two planes, rotating sprays are typically non-directional. This results in the distribution of equal quantities of cleaning solutions in all directions, thus requiring that all surfaces receive the cleaning solution flow rate and pressure necessary to remove residuals from the most difficult area(s) of the equipment being cleaned, and this can cause inefficiencies in solution usage. Rotating spray devices typically spray two points at a time within the equipment being cleaned, thus requiring a minimum time period (often 7–10 minutes) for complete contact of all surfaces with cleaning solutions.

Rotating spray devices are typically fabricated of stainless steel and non-stainless steel parts of non-hygienic design. They are typically not intended for product contact or permanent installation processing vessels and equipment, thus requiring installation prior to and removal following cleaning.

The cleaning solution flow rate required to clean vessels using rotating spray devices is often less than that for fixed-type sprays because of the added physical cleaning done by impingement. However, a significant portion of the cleaning solution flow reduction due to impingement can be lost because of the non-directional pattern of most rotating sprays. Since rotating spray devices are designed to clean surfaces by physical (impingement) and chemical means, they typically require supply pressures of 60–100 psig, which is relatively high. Rotating spray devices are often less reliable and require more maintenance than fixed-type sprays because they have moving parts and their spray patterns can be adversely affected by small to moderate variations in supply pressure. These characteristics make rotating spray devices more difficult to validate than fixed-type sprays.

Because rotating spray devices can provide a moderate to high degree of impingement, very tenacious residues may be more easily removed than with fixed-type sprays. However, this is not typically significant for biopharmaceutical equipment cleaning.

CLEANING AGENT DOSING METHODS AND EQUIPMENT

Automatic cleaning systems require the automated addition of cleaning agents for reliable and repeatable operation. The selection of appropriate methods and equipment for cleaning agent addition is based upon several factors and these are as follows.

Common Methods of Cleaning Agent Addition

There are several commonly used methods for the automatic addition of cleaning agents. The selection of an appropriate method often depends upon the configuration of the cleaning system. The following is a brief description of the three most common methods and their likely applications.

Constant Feed Systems

Constant feed cleaning agent addition systems, as their name implies, add cleaning agent(s) continuously and at a constant rate to the cleaning solution as it flows to the equipment being cleaned during wash steps of the cleaning cycle. This method is most often used with non-recirculating systems as the return flow is sent to drain, and thus the supply flow is always "fresh water." These systems often have much higher usage rates of cleaning agents than systems that recirculate.

Conductivity Based Systems

Conductivity based cleaning agent addition systems use conductivity sensing instruments to determine when cleaning agent addition equipment should be operated to maintain a setpoint level of cleaner within a wash solution storage tank(s). This method is most often used with multi-tank re-use systems that recirculate washing solutions and have separate tanks for the make-up and storage of washing solutions.

"Known Volume" Based Systems

"Known volume" based cleaning agent addition systems add cycle specific quantities of cleaners to the cleaning solutions during wash steps in a cleaning cycle. The amount of cleaning agent added is based upon the desired concentration and the quantity of water in the circuit, which is the "known volume." This method is typically used with single-use systems that recirculate washing solutions.

Commonly Used Cleaning Agent Addition Equipment

Cleaning agent addition to cleaning solutions most often involves the pumping of liquid cleaner(s) into a flowing stream or liquid in a cleaning solution storage tank. The most commonly used pumping methods for cleaning agent addition are discussed below.

Diaphragm Pumps

Air and electrically driven diaphragm pumps are quite often used for the automatic addition of cleaning agents to cleaning solutions. These are typically positive displacement pumps fabricated of corrosion resistant stainless steel or plastic materials. They are capable of dosing precise quantities of liquid cleaners into storage tanks or solution streams of relatively high pressures, and diaphragm pumps are capable of a wide range of flow rates. The most significant problems with these pumps are that they can be hard to prime and cleaning agents can be siphoned through them if external anti-siphon devices are not added to the cleaning agent dosing system.

Peristaltic Pumps

Electrically driven peristaltic pumps are used for the automatic addition of cleaning agents to cleaning solutions. These are typically positive displacement pumps which rely on the deformation of an elastomer tube for the pumping of cleaning agents. They are capable of dosing precise quantities of liquid cleaners into the storage tank's solution streams of relatively high pressures, but peristaltic pumps are not capable of as wide a range of flow rates as other types of pumps. The most significant problem with these pumps are that the elastomer tubing that they use requires frequent replacement due to fatigue, and they have relatively low flow rate capabilities as compared with some of the other pumps.

Piston Pumps

Air driven piston pumps are used for the automatic addition of cleaning agents to cleaning solutions. These are typically positive displacement pumps which are fabricated of a mix of corrosion resistant and non-corrosion resistant materials. They are capable of dosing precise quantities of liquid cleaners into storage tanks or solution streams of relatively high pressures, but piston pumps are not capable of as wide a range of flow rates as other types of pumps. The most significant problems with these pumps are corrosion of non-stainless parts, a fairly narrow range of flow rates, potential for siphoning, and they do not have flow rate capabilities as high as some of the other pumps.

Gear Pumps

Electrically driven gear pumps are used for the automatic addition of cleaning agents to cleaning solutions. These are typically positive displacement rotary pumps which are fabricated of corrosion resistant materials. They are capable of dosing fairly precise quantities of liquid cleaners into storage tanks or solution streams of relatively high pressures and gear pumps are capable of a wide a range of flow rates. The most significant problems with these pumps are that they can be very hard to prime, cleaning agents can be siphoned through them if external anti-siphon devices are not added to the cleaning agent dosing system, and they require a higher degree of maintenance than the other types of pumps.

Venturi Feeders

While not a pump, a venturi feeder can draw cleaning agent(s) into a solution stream via the vacuum generated by the solution stream flowing through its nozzle. They are capable of a fairly narrow range of flow rates and their "pumping rate" changes with changes in the solution flow rate through the venturi nozzle. This may hurt the repeatability of the device as compared with the other pumps discussed in this section. The major advantage of venturi feeders is that they have no moving parts and are very simple to operate and maintain.

CLEAN-OUT-OF-PLACE SYSTEMS AND OTHER CLEANING EQUIPMENT

While CIP systems are responsible for much of the cleaning done in biopharmaceutical facilities, semi-automatic and manual cleaning is also commonplace. Clean-out-of-place (COP) systems and other parts washing equipment are often used to clean miscellaneous fittings and parts. These types of systems are described below.

COP Systems and Parts Washers

COP systems typically consist of a single open tank used for rinsing and washing operations, a water supply valve, a steam supply valve, a drain valve and a recirculation pump. These systems may be completely manual or they may include a cleaning agent feed system, instrumentation for recording and control, and a control system.

Small parts and fittings are cleaned in a COP system by loading the pieces to be cleaned into a rack in the COP tank, filling the COP tank with water, and starting the recirculation pump. This rinses the items being cleaned, and on some systems there is constant water addition and discharge during the rinses to try to carry as much residue as possible out of the system prior to the Alkali

Wash step of the cycle. Following this first rinse, the recirculation pump is stopped, the tank is drained and refilled with water, and the recirculation pump is re-started. The steam valve is then opened to heat the solution, cleaning agent(s) are added, and the hot alkaline washing solution is recirculated for a preset time. When the alkaline wash is complete, the steam valve is closed, the recirculation pump is stopped, the tank is again drained and refilled with water, and the recirculation pump is re-started. This rinses residual alkaline cleaner from the parts being cleaned, and depending upon the requirements of the system, may be repeated several times. An acid wash step followed by a final rinse may also be used.

Some or all of the sequence described above may be done manually or automatically depending upon the control capability of the COP system. The types of parts that may reasonably be washed in a COP system are typically those whose geometries enable the flow of cleaning solutions through or completely around them. The configuration of parts placement within the COP tank may present challenges in operation and validation alike in insuring that turbulent solution has contacted all surfaces of the items being cleaned.

Other types of parts washers, such as ultrasonic cleaners, are used in the biopharmaceutical industry. The operation of these types of devices is typically unique to specific manufacturers and often manual. The validation of this equipment should be based upon the same types of criteria used for CIP and COP systems.

Glassware Washers

Because many biopharmaceutical processes require glass containers and other parts, glassware washers are often used. These can be configured in many ways including single door units where dirty and clean items are loaded and unloaded through a single door, and "pass through" units where dirty items are loaded through one door and clean items are unloaded through another door on the opposite side. Most washers have a single chamber with a rack that hold the glassware. The dirty items are loaded onto spindles, and water is sprayed through the spindles to clean the items. Glassware washers may be manually operated or they may have a fairly high degree of automation. In either case, glassware washing is typically a "batch operation."

Many different cleaning cycles and variations are used for washing glassware. For biopharmaceutical glassware, most washers use DI or WFI water, or a progressive cycle where the highest quality water is used for the last step(s) of the cleaning cycle. Because the residues on the glassware may be proteinaceous, many washers use an alkaline cleaning agent in addition to water for cleaning, and some may also have an acid rinse step. Washing glassware at elevated temperatures (60–80°C) is not uncommon.

Vial and Stopper Washers

Vial and stopper cleaning is important in biopharmaceutical manufacturing as most products are parenterals. Their proper operation is critical as they clean the final product container.

Vial washers are often used to remove soluble contaminants, particulates, and to perform depyrogenation of the glass. Vial washers may be of batch or continuous design and their cycles are often short in duration. A typical vial washing cycle may consist of alternating cleaning solution and compressed air streams. The cleaning solution might be WFI, DI and WFI, or detergent and WFI. Vial washing is often done at elevated or alternating hot and cold temperatures.

Stopper washers are typically used for the same purposes as vial washer, that is the removal of soluble contaminants and particulates, and depyrogenation. There are several types of stopper washers in common use including impingement, overflow and rotating drum machines. Impingement washers hold the stoppers in a rack and clean them with a high pressure spray. Overflow washers clean the stoppers by immersing them in a cleaning liquid and agitating them with compressed nitrogen. Rotating drum washers clean the stoppers by spinning them in a drum filled with a cleaning liquid. Many stopper washing cycles are used depending upon the type of washing equipment and desired result (e.g., depyrogenation, siliconization, etc.). Stopper washing is often done at elevated temperatures.

SUMMARY

The cleaning of processing equipment in the biopharmaceutical industry is accomplished by systems of many different designs and with varying degrees of automation. It is important that the cleaning strategies and equipment are appropriately applied to the equipment being cleaned, the residues being removed, and the operational constraints of the facility in which they will operate. The challenges involved in the validation of these systems may vary, but it is critical that the basic design, sequence of operation, instrumentation, control system, and cleaning agent feed equipment are well understood by those responsible for their start-up, validation, and operation.

Section II

VALIDATION CONCEPTS

The previous section explored the process of designing cleanable equipment, cleaning systems and cleaning mechanisms. This section draws upon the foundation laid in the previous chapters and looks at the mechanisms used to verify that the cleaning process is effective and reliable. The techniques used to provide the assurance that a process is performing acceptably are generally known as *validation*.

Section II presents methods that can be used to plan, prepare for, and execute a cleaning validation study. Chapter 4, "Validation Study Design," begins the section by identifying the basic components of a validation study and takes the reader through the process of developing the test documentation that can be used to verify that a cleaning process is effective and consistent. The key to a successful cleaning study relies heavily upon the sampling and analytical methods used to determine cleanliness. Chapter 5, "Sampling Methods," analyzes the currently used sampling methods for cleaning validation in the biotechnology industry. Included are descriptions of the methods, typical applications and examples of sampling procedures. Rinse water, visual examination, surface sampling techniques and recovery studies are presented and discussed. Because sampling techniques are inherently dependent on the nature of the process and equipment being tested, their impact on the development of a validation strategy is important to recognize.

Chapter 6, "Analytical Methods Which Support Cleaning Validation Studies," provides the corresponding piece of the testing puzzle to sampling technology—*analytical methods*. Analytical methods used for cleaning validation range from the simple (pH) to the complex (product specific assays). This broad spectrum is further complicated by the new advances in testing technology being applied to the problems being encountered. Total Organic Carbon (TOC) for example is a promising technology that, while not new in the testing world per se, is now beginning to be applied to the evaluation of cleaning effectiveness. Testing to demonstrate cleanliness is a difficult a challenge to engineering and scientific abilities. Frequently one is looking for trace amounts of a soil for which assay sensitivity may be limited. Inhibition or interaction with the sampling method itself can often cause problems and must be carefully considered when selecting an analytical method. For these reasons, Chapter 6 (like Chapter 5) is crucial for those developing cleaning validation strategies.

In the end it all comes down to the oft asked question "How clean is clean?" Chapter 7 does not answer the question, nor for that matter can this book. Chapter 7, "Approaches to Establishing Cleaning Validation Acceptance Criteria," does, however, provide as much information as is currently available on the subject of determining acceptable levels of residues for biotechnology processes. This issue is particularly pertinent to the biotechnology industry where the contaminant(s) may, for multiproduct facilities, be a final drug product itself. The traditional methodologies for determining acceptable limits for contaminants is complicated in the biotechnology industry by the fact that the final drug product, often a complex protein, may be detectable only by assays requiring a fully active protein, rarely the situation following most cleaning processes, which are designed to denature proteins.

Section II provides the latest information available on the subject of biotechnology cleaning validation emphasizing process validation study design, sampling and analytical methods, and acceptance criteria.

An example of a cleaning process validation protocol is presented in the Appendix at the end of this book to further aid in the development of a validation study.

4

Validation Study Design

The validation of a cleaning process, like the validation of most manufacturing processes, is performed as a series of sequential steps. Each step should add value to the cleaning process, building upon the value of the previous step. When complete, these steps should provide documented evidence demonstrating that the cleaning process is capable of effective, consistent operation. This chapter focuses upon the current approaches used to validate cleaning systems and processes in the biopharmaceutical industry.

Demonstrating cleaning *consistency* is accomplished by verifying that a system has the capability to perform an operation or process and then verifying repeatable system performance. This typically involves verifying that each piece of the system is installed properly, operates as intended, is programmed properly, and can effectively duplicate its intended operation. These steps are similar to those used in most validation studies and are presented in this chapter in the same logical flow using examples and case studies when ever possible.

The concept of cleaning consistency is then combined with the concept of cleaning *effectiveness*. A discussion of Process Validation explains how to provide evidence that a cleaning process effectively performs its intended operation using industry examples and presents a discussion of commonly applied strategies. This section is the major emphasis of the chapter as it is often the most difficult and time consuming effort of a cleaning validation program.

THE VALIDATION SEQUENCE

The sequential approach used for the validation of a cleaning system and/or process is not unlike the approaches used for the validation of most processing systems. In this sequence, the first step is typically the development of a Master Plan or section of a Master Plan. The plan is used to give direction and illustrate when, where, how and why, cleaning validation activities are to take place.

Master Plans typically identify the Installation Qualification (IQ) and Operational Qualification (OQ) testing that will be used to assure both the process equipment and the cleaning equipment operate as they were designed prior to testing the cleaning process for effectiveness. It is important that both process equipment and cleaning system equipment are initially qualified prior to initiating cleaning *process* validation as the proper operation of the process equipment is often as critical (in terms of cleaning) as that of the cleaning equipment itself.

The final step in the validation sequence is also typically the most challenging and involves the verification of the cleaning process consistency and efficacy. Process validation is the step in which cleaning effectiveness and reliability are challenged and compared against pre-determined acceptance criteria.

Master Plan

Master Plans are often thought of in terms of defining the overall validation plan for an entire manufacturing facility and its associated equipment. The concepts embodied within a Master Plan are however, useful to the development of a successful cleaning validation program and can be used to create a "cleaning master plan."

A cleaning master plan can be used to define how cleaning is accomplished and why, and the approach that will be used to demonstrate that the cleaning is consistently effective. The scope of the plan should be defined first. Clean-in-place (CIP), clean-out-of-place (COP), automated packaged washers, and manual cleaning may all be covered in one plan or separate plans as appropriate. The plan should briefly describe the equipment and process steps used to operate the manufacturing process. Often, steps are chosen or created based upon the logical "breaks" in the process with cleaning procedures for each step being described along with details of the process and an analysis of the anticipated residues for the specific step. The plan should provide a list of the pertinent raw materials used in the production process, the materials of product contact and the anticipated cleaning agents.

Once the plan has defined the equipment, the process and the cleaning procedures used to clean the process equipment, the goals of the cleaning process should be clearly stated. In some cases, goals may vary for different steps in the manufacturing process. The goal for instance in an upstream process or non-critical area may be to remove all residues to below visible detection while the goal for a final purification step may be more stringent.

When the goals of the cleaning program are defined, the testing procedures needed to qualify or validate that the goals are successfully achieved should be discussed. Testing procedures should be related to each goal to correlate testing with expected results. A cleaning validation master plan should also identify what will be done to qualify the cleaning system itself. Typically, this would be an identification of the IQ and OQ work that will be used to verify the proper installation and operation of the cleaning system.

Whether this form of planning information is contained in a master plan specific to cleaning validation, a facility validation master plan, or other documentation, it is important that the information be agreed upon, written down and understood by those groups affected.

Installation Qualification of a Cleaning System

Installation Qualification (IQ) is the process used to verify and document that a given system has been installed properly and that the components within the system comply with manufacturer's installation and design specifications, cGMPs, and appropriate codes [1]. The installation qualification may include but is not limited to the following:

- System Description

- Component Descriptions and Materials of Construction

- Materials in Contact With Product

- Instrument List

- Safety Requirements

- Utility Requirement Description

- Listing of Appropriate SOPs

- Listings and Locations of Drawings, Manuals and Specifications

- Comparison of installed system to specifications, drawings and requirements for verification of proper installation and documentation

- Software Configuration Management

The value of an IQ can be enhanced if it is tailored to fit the needs of the company. If an IQ is going to be used in a start-up situation for instance, the IQ can serve as a useful checking procedure to verify the accuracy of the associated P&IDs. The IQ can serve to verify that all instrumentation, specified for the system was installed where it was supposed to be and has been appropriately tagged or labeled.

The IQ can be developed as a formal validation protocol or in some cases may be included as part of a vendor supplied turn-over package. If supplied by the vendor, the IQ should be verified by the users as they have the ultimate responsibility for the system.

Operational Qualification of a Cleaning System

Operational Qualification (OQ) testing is used to verify and document that the cleaning system operates according to design requirements and specifications. OQ testing is critical because it establishes the ability of the cleaning system to deliver and/or circulate cleaning solutions according to preset circuit specific parameters including: flow rates, chemical concentrations, temperatures, pressures, etc. A well planned OQ will reduce the likelihood of process validation failure due to equipment malfunction or improper operation.

An important consideration when performing an OQ on a CIP system is that the cleaning circuit wash/rinse times (developed and tested during the OQ stage of the validation process) may need to be changed as a result of the OQ testing. Cycle development work is often performed just prior to process validation. Cycle parameters that are commonly adjusted include rinse cycle times or volumes and cleaning agent concentration. Consequently, the OQ should be designed to cover a variety of final operational possibilities. This can be done by testing operational functions over a range of operating conditions. For example, verifying that a Supply Pump Time On parameter operates successfully over a programmable range of 0 to 99 minutes provides assurance that any future changes to the parameter within the tested range will function properly.

Because OQs are typically executed following system installation and prior to normal operational use, they also provide an ideal environment to collect useful operational data about the system. For example, a parameter such as the time required for cleaning solution heating can be recorded during OQ testing. Even though the parameter may not be critical, the information may be used later for cycle development or system performance evaluation.

The following is a review of areas of focus for operational qualification testing of cleaning systems.

Calibration Verification

Prior to actual OQ testing, all critical instruments should be calibrated. The importance of this seemingly insignificant step cannot be over emphasized. If instruments critical to the operation of the system have not been calibrated then data collected during the subsequent OQ and process validation steps may be invalid.

Cleaning System Operational Sequence

A cleaning cycle or program is typically comprised of a series of steps performed in a pre-defined sequence. Verification of the operational sequence should assure that the cleaning system cycle(s) operates as intended. This functional testing should include verification that the cycle steps are executed in the correct order, confirmation that for each cycle step the proper operation of system components (such as valves, pumps, instruments, etc.) occurs, and verification that the design intent of the cleaning system is realized (e.g., vessels are drained at the end of drain steps, etc.).

Verification of a cleaning program sequence can be as simple as the manual observation of the cleaning system's operation (such as sequence step indicator, valve positioning) during sequence execution. This exercise should be performed at least once for each different program the cleaning system executes. Examples of different programs might include one for cleaning vessels, another for cleaning process lines, another for rinsing only, and so on. This does not mean that the program for each *circuit* must be verified as it is common for several circuits to use the same cleaning program with different cleaning process parameters (such as flow rates, temperatures, rinse times, etc.), rather, each cleaning system program with a different logic sequence should be verified to assure proper operation.

> Example 4:1: Verify that cleaning program 1 (Large Tank Cleaning) executes in the following sequence: Pre-rinse, Hot Caustic Wash, Rinse, Hot Acid Wash, Rinse, Rinse, Air Dry. Accomplish verification by initiating the program and determining that the step indicators for each step light in the proper sequence as defined in the cleaning sequence specification document.

The verification of the proper operation of cleaning system components in each cleaning cycle step is of equal importance to the overall operational qualification. As with the cycle sequence step execution verification, consistent operation of the cleaning system components during each cleaning cycle sequence step is crucial to repeatable cleaning results. Verification is usually accomplished by visual inspection of the system components (such as valves, pumps, instruments, etc.) for proper operation per their prescribed cleaning sequence step during cleaning cycle execution. Such verification can help identify miswired valves or components. This work should also be performed on a "per program" basis.

> Example 4.2: Verify that the system components operate properly and in sequence for cleaning program 2 (Media Prep Line and Tank Cleaning) Accomplish verification by initiating the program and examining the valve actuator indicators, verify that each of the cleaning circuit valves opens and closes properly and in the proper sequence.

Critical cleaning process parameters

Virtually all CIP systems control the cleaning process by modifying one or more of several critical process parameters. The most common parameters controlled during CIP operation are time, temperature, concentration and flow rate. Depending on the system and its configuration, each of these critical parameters will most likely require testing as part of the OQ study.

> **Time**   Time is the most common and most frequently modified cleaning parameter in a CIP cleaning circuit. Often, each step of a cleaning cycle is time dependent. A typical cleaning cycle for example may have a 10-minute wash step followed by a 5-minute drain step, followed by three 5-minute rinse steps. OQ testing should verify the accuracy and the reliability of the time parameters because these parameters are directly related to cleaning effectiveness.

> **Temperature**   Cleaning agents are often heated to increase the effectiveness of the cleaning process. Because the heating process often is dependent on a number of potentially variable parameters (starting solution temperature, utility supply temperature (if heat energy is supplied by steam for example), it is important to test the temperature control process during the OQ. Testing should verify, if possible, that adequate temperature control is maintained under normal load and maximum anticipated load conditions.

> **Cleaning Agent Concentration**   Cleaning agent concentration has a direct impact on cleaning effectiveness. Too little cleaning agent can result in failure to reduce process residues, while too much cleaning agent can result in cleaning agent residue removal problems. The addition and consequent concentration of the cleaning agents that are used may be controlled automatically or manually. Regardless of the method of addition testing should be performed to verify that the proper concentration of cleaning agents is reliably achieved.

> **Flow Rate**   The volumetric flow rate of liquids through production equipment (tanks, piping, etc.) can affect cleaning efficacy and hence should also be examined during OQ testing. To assure that cleaning solution is in contact with the entire interior surface of a pipe for example, the minimum flow rate required to coat the interior surface of the pipe may be calculated from the size of the pipe and the properties of the fluid. The system can then be tested during the OQ to verify that the minimum flow rate is achieved.

Cleaning Solution Surface Contact

If sprayballs are used to deliver cleaning solution to equipment surfaces, spray patterns can be checked to assure adequate cleaning agent coverage. One commonly used method is to coat equipment surfaces with an innocuous cleanable marker. Common markers include aqueous solutions of riboflavin or powdered milk. After the markers or dyes are pumped through a sprayball, the equipment is then visually inspected to assure complete coverage. This method can also help identify possible surface sampling sites for later process validation studies if hard to clean areas are located. It should be realized that cleaning solution contact does not necessarily correlate to effective cleaning, however it can be important in the overall analysis of the effectiveness of the cleaning program.

CLEANING PROCESS VALIDATION (PV)

Building upon the foundation established by the IQ and OQ, process validation is the step in the cleaning validation program where actual cleaning processes are challenged and tested for effectiveness and consistency. Typically, a cleaning process validation study requires the development of a test protocol, execution of the protocol, analysis of data, and the establishment of conclusions based on this data. It is the development and execution of the protocol that are frequently the most time consuming tasks and hence the area of focus for the remainder of this chapter.

The development of an effective cleaning validation protocol requires careful analysis of several factors—the manufacturing process, the biochemistry of the product, equipment design, and potential validation testing strategies. The analysis of these topics typically is performed simultaneously as each is dependent upon the other.

Analysis of each stage of the manufacturing process is used to help identify the general and specific goals of the cleaning process. The manufacturing process must be examined to determine what kind of processing activity is occurring. Does the process inherently contain many types of potential contaminants such as in a fermentation step, or are there relatively few such as in a formulation or filling step? What are the materials/products going into the process? Other questions that may be asked when analyzing the process focus on the cleaning methodology itself. For instance, is the cleaning process manual, clean-out-of-place, clean-in-place or a combination of each? The information obtained from the review of the manufacturing process and related cleaning regimen can then be used to help identify appropriate sampling methods, analytical methods, and acceptance criteria.

Once the process and product have been analyzed and the information used to help determine the role of a given cleaning process, a validation testing strategy can be developed. Validation strategies are typically selected based upon the criticality of the cleaning process. Ranging from relatively simple–normal operational process testing, to complex–worst case testing, these strategies require significantly different validation approaches.

Process, Product, and Contaminant Considerations

Ultimately, acceptance criteria specific to individual sampling and testing methods are established based on possible contamination scenarios and perceived process sensitivity to potential contaminants. The establishment of these criteria is based on the ability to determine what the actual contaminants are and to what degree they need to be removed. Information that will aid in making these decisions can be gathered by studying how a process works biochemically and how the related equipment works mechanically. One must also consider how contamination problems may impact the ability to control process parameters and product quality [2].

Several biopharmaceutical areas where these principles can be applied are discussed below. Emphasis is placed on evaluating potential problems from contamination of trace amounts of residuals at these stages.

Fermentation/Cell Culture Operations

Fermentation and/or cell culture processing steps are initially used to grow recombinant cells in a growth promoting media under controlled environmental conditions to a desired density. Once the optimal density is reached the cells are induced to synthesize the desired biological product. Ultimately, these steps also result in the production of thousands of other organic substances, some or all of which can be considered potential contaminants to the current processing stage or to processing stages further downstream [3]. Besides these biological contaminants, other additives such as antibiotics, antifoam, cleaning agents, media, salts, and vitamins, also have the potential to contaminate the next production batch.

Recognizing that fermentation/cell culture operations often produce an endless number of possible contaminants, deciding what these contaminants can potentially do to the next production batch becomes the crux of the cleaning validation problem. Contaminants can potentially affect a wide range of process parameters. In the fermentation or cell culture process examples of processes or specific parameters that could be affected by contaminants include:

- Growth rates

- Cell induction

- Downstream purification

- Sterilization efficacy

- Mechanical operations

One way to determine the potential effect of residual contamination is to review the optimal conditions that need to exist to promote cell growth and induction. If there is a probability that trace amounts of a contaminant (such as residual cleaning agents, concentrated acids or bases, etc.) could adversely affect these conditions, the testing strategy should incorporate specific analytical methods that would detect such contaminants. Detection of such contaminants can help protect downstream purification operations from producing unexpectedly low product yields due to inadequate cleaning regimes.

When evaluating the impact of a potential contaminant on a fermentation/ cell culture step, downstream purification operations must also be considered. If cellular components can be shown to be cleared downstream, then potentially less emphasis can be placed on these contaminants.

Another primary concern when dealing with fermentation or cell culture cleaning processes is the impact cleaning has on the efficacy of the associated sterilization procedures. Soil that remains after cleaning could adversely affect sterilization by preventing steam penetration or chemical contact. Fermentation and cell culture equipment are especially susceptible to this problem due to the nature of the operations themselves.

Often, fermentation operations do not place the equipment surfaces in direct contact with the desired product protein. This is due to the encapsulation of the product by the host organism. As such, the issues of product cross-contamination and multiproduct manufacturing are considered to be of less concern than for the later stages of processing and cleaning emphasis is directed at removing residues that are potentially harmful to the host organism.

Recovery and Purification Operations

Purification processes typically isolate the desired biological product either mechanically by centrifugation, homogenization, or filtration, or chemically by precipitation or chromatography. Each purification step separates the desired biological product from impurities or contaminants in the process stream. Typically, the number and concentration of potential contaminants decreases with each subsequent purification step.

Recognizing the potential contaminants at each step of the process, and evaluating how such residuals could affect future processing will facilitate meaningful validation studies. In purification operations examples of process parameters that could be affected include:

- Final product purity
- Product yields
- Mechanical operations

Recovery stages of purification (i.e., filtration, cell disruption, centrifugation) typically contact different types of contaminants than column-based purification steps. This is important to recognize when establishing a testing scheme and when determining appropriate acceptance criteria. Column chromatography operations are more likely to be affected by slight changes in process conditions such as pH or conductivity, or by other trace contamination than fermentation or recovery steps.

If purification equipment is to be used for multiproduct operations, the associated validation testing scheme and acceptance criteria will need to reflect the possibility that each product could contaminate the next product campaign. Rinse water, visual inspection, and/or surface samples can be taken to prove that residual product is not building up in the equipment and that the product is removed to the degree deemed necessary to allow for multiproduct use. Once the product has been sufficiently isolated and purified, normal product specification testing will verify product purity and should provide further evidence that cleaning procedures are effective.

Formulation/Filling Operations

The final manufacturing steps consist of formulating and filling the desired product. Functionally and chemically these steps are straightforward, yet from a cleaning validation perspective they are considered the most critical. Contamination resulting from inadequate cleaning at this stage in the manufacturing process has the highest probability of affecting final product purity or final product concentration. Because formulation and filling equipment frequently are used with multiple products at their highest purity, inadequate cleaning at this step introduces the greatest possibility for cross-contamination.

Careful attention to the chemistry of the cleaning process at this stage is important. The biologically active components that are present prior to cleaning will most likely be denatured or otherwise inactivated during the cleaning process. This leaves a challenging set of circumstances when evaluating or determining a relevant testing scheme. It may be impractical, for example, to demonstrate that active ingredients do not remain after cleaning because their residue may be difficult or even impossible to detect depending on the detection methods used. Therefore, consideration should be given to testing that can detect inactive biological residue (i.e., SDS-PAGE testing for rinse water, or Total Organic Carbon testing for either rinse water or surfaces).

Manual Cleaning

Manual cleaning processes pose an additional validation challenge. The challenge is to demonstrate that a manual process is consistent given operator performance differences. In this case the cleaning validation program should focus on providing evidence that each cleaning procedure is effective using different operators and that a well documented training program is in place to ensure different operators clean consistently. Often validation documentation is combined with periodic verification testing to provide evidence of process effectiveness and consistency.

Equipment Considerations

Once the process and product considerations have been carefully examined, the next step is to determine when, how, and where to perform sampling for analysis and visual inspection. Three aspects that can be evaluated to aid in these decisions are equipment design, materials of construction, and the type of cleaning methods that will be used.

The design of a piece of equipment affects its ability to be cleaned and tested [4]. Often for example, the equipment design precludes certain testing schemes such as visual inspection or surface sampling by nature of surface inaccessibility. Careful review of the equipment design will frequently aid in determining where and how to sample process equipment. Additionally, a thorough review of the equipment design can identify potential areas for contaminant build-up and sampling sites, thereby strengthening the associated validation study. For example, a port in the top dome of a tank may be difficult to clean due to a problem with the associated spray pattern of the cleaning agents during cleaning. This port could be targeted as a specific sampling site and used to potentially represent a worst case cleaning location.

The materials that are used to construct manufacturing equipment can also affect the ability to clean the equipment. Product, process residue, and cleaning agents will react with different types of surfaces with different affinities. Reviewing the materials used to construct manufacturing equipment will aid in determining where to take cleaning validation samples. Porous materials, for example, may have a greater probability of retaining soils than less porous materials and consequently may serve as hard to clean locations for use as sampling sites.

Review of the cleaning process, whether manual or automated, will complete the equipment analysis picture and help determine when and where to take samples. For a system cleaned by CIP, rinse samples can be taken downstream of the last process piping or in the bottom-most outlet of a vessel being cleaned. The samples can be taken either during the final rinse to verify that soluble residues have been removed or throughout the cycle to demonstrate an actual reduction of soil.

When working with a manual cleaning process the sampling process becomes slightly more complex. Deciding where to take samples depends heavily upon the equipment geometry. Deciding how and when to take samples depends on the size of the equipment and how the equipment is rinsed. Equipment that can be reassembled to contain liquids (i.e., portable tank, or filling line) can be rinsed with purified water or Water for Injection (WFI), and samples collected and tested. Other miscellaneous equipment can be rinsed into a sterile sample container. Taking rinse samples from a sink is also an option although it complicates the information due to the fact that the samples contact more that just product contact surfaces.

VALIDATION TESTING STRATEGIES

A validation testing strategy should be planned, agreed upon, and most importantly be practical. Far too often, needlessly complicated and expensive testing scenarios are created that challenge systems in ways for which they were never designed to perform. A good validation testing strategy will address those issues that are important to the *consistent, effective* performance of the cleaning process. As a minimum, this should include *normal process testing* to verify that under normal, controlled conditions, the cleaning process is effective.

Depending on the results of the analysis of the process, the product and the equipment, testing strategies may be expanded or combined to include conditions that while not considered "normal," may occur during processing. *Edge of failure* and *range testing* are strategies that can be used to expand upon *normal process testing*. While rarely practical, for certain situations *worst case* testing may be an appropriate cleaning validation strategy. Worst case testing challenges the cleaning process with conditions that are not expected to occur during normal operations. A review of each of these testing strategies is provided below:

Normal Process Testing

The most common, and certainly the most straightforward testing strategy, normal process testing (or performance testing) verifies that when operated under "normal" conditions, the cleaning process is consistent and effective. Normal process testing relies heavily upon the demonstration that the process is in a state of control and does not vary from run to run or cycle to cycle. In order to justify the use of normal process testing for a validation testing strategy, the "normal" conditions and parameters should be well documented in the operational procedures governing the cleaning of the equipment.

If a cleaning procedure is itself highly variable, then normal process testing may not be sufficient to assure the cleaning process is effective or reliable. For example, if the operational procedures specify that a cleaning circuit is to have a pre-rinse duration of between 10 and 20 minutes, normal operational testing may only cover part of the rinse duration range and hence not be capable of assuring that a 10-minute or 20-minute pre-rinse duration is effective.

Edge of Failure

By modifying cleaning process parameters to induce cleaning failure one can determine the "edge of failure" for the specific parameter. For example, by decreasing the final rinse time of a cleaning cycle until the end of rinse pH sample fails, one can determine (approximately) when the edge of failure occurs for rinsing as it relates to pH. Once the edge of failure has been determined, the operating parameters associated with the cleaning method can be adjusted to provide a "safety factor" thereby providing assurance that a cleaning process is effective. Example cleaning parameters that may be adjusted to establish the edge of failure include:

- Cleaning Solution and Rinse Water Temperatures
- Cleaning Solution and Rinse Water Volumes
- Cleaning Solution and Rinse Water Flow Rates
- Cleaning Solution Concentrations
- Extended Hold Times Prior to Cleaning
- Contact Times

Example 4.3: Verify that for a specific CIP cycle sufficient rinsing action occurs so that a basic cleaning agent is removed: Samples are taken at 1-minute intervals throughout the final rinse circuit from a return to CIP Port and analyzed for pH. Once the edge of failure has been established, the circuit is adjusted to assure adequate rinsing.

Range Testing

Like most validated processes, cleaning processes are typically operated within specific physical ranges (temperature, pressure, cleaning agent concentration, hold or rinse times, etc.). In order to account for cleaning parameter ranges, validation strategies often "force" parameter(s) to their upper and lower limits. This range testing approach provides additional assurance that for a given cleaning procedure, the process is effective and reliable over the entire parameter range.

Consideration of the total number of variable cleaning parameters is important to prevent the testing of an infinite combination of range testing scenarios. A reasonable approach based on range testing *critical* parameters should be employed. Properly designed experiments can reduce the number of runs required to test these parameters. Critical parameters can be determined based upon information gained from the analysis of the process, the equipment and the product as described previously.

Worst Case Testing

Just as range testing is an expansion of *normal process testing*, worst case testing expands upon the range testing strategy. Conceptually, worst case validation testing strategies are used to reduce the total quantity of validation studies for a system or process. The concept is relatively straightforward—by demonstrating that the cleaning process is consistent and effective for the worst case conditions, all other conditions are by default assured of consistent, effective operation. The difficulty and reason this approach is rarely used for cleaning validation, is that because of the number of variable parameters that exist for cleaning processes, it is often more difficult to identify the "worst case conditions" than it is to validate several normal processes or apply a reasonable range testing strategy.

Worst case testing can be an effective validation strategy in certain multiproduct situations. If a worst case product can be determined, surface interaction and or solubility for example, then that material could be used as a worst case challenge material for multiproduct cleaning validation studies. In so doing, one can eliminate the need to repeat cleaning studies on all pieces of equipment each time a new product is introduced as long as the new product has been shown to be more soluble or less interactive than the worst case material.

While often impractical as a common cleaning validation strategy, worst case testing does have its place and can be useful if carefully applied. Spiking studies, for example, can be used to demonstrate that a process step is effective at removing a cross-contaminating product introduced upstream of the step.

As with range testing strategies, worst case testing can be combined with other strategies to provide a comprehensive and effective validation approach. Examples of worst case testing parameters that may be included in such an approach include:

- Product in highest concentration
- Product in the hardest to clean locations
- Product on the hardest to clean surface
- Material from the "dirtiest" stage of the process

Equipment Preparation Issues

Another factor to consider when examining process cleaning procedures and practices is to view them in light of all of the activities that take place in order to prepare equipment for manufacturing. Cleaning procedures are often used to prepare equipment for sterilization or sanitization. If cleaning procedures are inadequate sterilization procedures may be ineffective or residues may be baked on to equipment surfaces. Samples can be taken after both cleaning and sterilization in order to develop an accurate view of the cleanliness of the equipment before manufacturing operations begin.

> Example 4.4: Verify that a filling line including tubing, connectors, and filling needles are cleaned effectively: Samples are taken after cleaning and sterilization. The filling line is assembled and a predetermined volume of rinse water is pumped through the filling apparatus. The rinse water is collected and sampled for residual product, Total Organic Carbon, microbial contaminants, and cleaning agents.

Testing of this nature can help ensure that the effects of the sterilization process and subsequent equipment reassembly are included in the cleaning validation.

SUMMARY

The process of validating cleaning procedures requires up–front investigation of the process that is to be cleaned. The purpose of this investigation is to aid in determining when, where, and why equipment needs to be sampled and tested. Studying the biochemistry of the process and related equipment design should help address these questions. Understanding current validation testing strategies and knowledge of current sampling techniques and available analytical detection methods will complete the picture. As each piece of the cleaning validation puzzle is completed, each system should be shown to provide consistent effective operation.

REFERENCES

1. Agalloco, J., *Validation of Aseptic Pharmaceutical Processes,* Dekker, 1986.

2. Berry, I.A., Nash, R.A., *Pharmaceutical process Validation*, Marcel Dekker, Inc., V57, 1993, pp 319–349.

3. Garnick, R., et al., "A Total Organic Carbon Analysis Method for Validating Cleaning between Products in Biopharmaceutical Manufacturing," Parenteral Drug Association, *Journal of parenteral Science and Technology,* V45(1), January/February, 1991, pp 13–19.

4. Jenkins, K.M., Vanderwielen, A.J., "Cleaning Validation: An Overall Perspective," *Pharmaceutical Technology,* 18:4, April 1994, pp 60–73.

5

Sampling Methods

The success or failure of any cleaning validation program is critically dependent upon the samples taken to evaluate cleaning effectiveness. Sampling methodologies vary tremendously depending on the nature of the equipment, the cleaning process, the product, and related soils. A sampling method that is highly successful for one operation in a plant may be inadequate for the next process step in the same manufacturing operation. This chapter focuses upon the sampling methods used most frequently for biotechnology cleaning validation studies.

Many sampling techniques can be used to obtain cleaning validation data. Visual inspection, solvent (water based) extraction, and surface sampling are common examples of sampling methods. Samples may be tested for specific residues or non-specific residues depending on the goals of the validation testing strategy.

Consider the soils commonly associated with the equipment when establishing a sampling program. If soils are water soluble, rinse water sampling can be used to demonstrate cleanliness. For insoluble soils, rinse water sampling may give false negative results and result in a need to use surface sampling techniques. Each major sampling method, its application and benefits and disadvantages is discussed in the following sections.

VISUAL INSPECTION

Visual inspection is probably the most effective qualitative method of determining equipment cleanliness due to the wide range of information that can be obtained from production equipment. Often soils that remain after cleaning can be seen at relatively low concentrations. In fact, most residues are visible at approximately 100 pg per 2" x 2" area [1].

Case Study 5.1

As part of a cleaning validation study, a bioreactor used in a multiproduct production operation was disassembled and visually inspected for residue after the bioreactor had been cleaned. It was noticed that the diaphragm of the media inlet valve was covered with a blackened residue. Further analysis indicated that the residue was media which had been baked onto the diaphragm by the steam used to sterilize the port after each use. Different media were used in this particular bioreactor due its use in multiproduct production operations and one media component from one product campaign was known to affect the growth rate of a different species of microorganism from a different product campaign also used in this bioreactor. Due to the possibility that this contamination may affect process control in one of the product campaigns, the diaphragm of the valve was replaced with a clean one and changed out between manufacturing campaigns. Due to the visual inspection portion in this particular cleaning validation study, the problem was detected and methods put in place to correct the situation.

RINSE WATER SAMPLING

Solvent extraction methods, such as rinse water sampling, are commonly used to determine equipment cleanliness [2]. Rinse water is probably the most commonly sampled element of a cleaning circuit due to the fact that rinse water is relatively easy to sample and is conducive to many analytical test methods. In a clean-in-place (CIP) cleaned system, rinse samples can be taken by installing a valve in the return to CIP line or from the lowest valve on the cleaned equipment. Solvents can be analyzed using a variety of testing methods including the following (each of which is discussed in detail in Chapter 6):

Residue Non–Specific Rinse Water Analytical Methods

- pH
- Conductivity
- Osmolarity

- Particle Counts

- Orthophosphate

- Total Microbial Count

- Total Organic Carbon

- Endotoxin Determination

- Total Dissolved Solids

- IR and UV Scans

- Absorbance

- USP Water Testing

Advantage: broad product application, standard methodology

Disadvantages: not product specific, potential analyte dilution effect

Residue Specific Rinse Water Analytical Methods

- Bioassays

- Immunoassays

- HPLC

- SDS-PAGE

- LAL

Advantage: product/active specific, frequently very quantitative to low levels
Disadvantage: methods must frequently be developed and validated for both product and degradation products, may be wide assay variability

Case Study 5.2

An automated cleaning circuit is used to clean a product dedicated transfer line connected to a formulation tank and a transfer panel in a filling suite. Formulated bulk is transferred through this line into the filling suite. The formulated bulk consists of protein, buffer, and a preservative, all of which are slightly soluble to soluble at pH 5–7 but very soluble at pH 2. The cleaning circuit includes a pre-rinse with purified water, a hot base (pH 10) and acid wash (pH 2), followed by a series of rinses with Water for Injection (WFI). Due to the configu-

(Continued on page 110)

(Continued from page 109)
ration of the transfer line and the inability to access the interior of the line, surface sampling was determined to be ineffective. Therefore, the sampling strategy was established solely on data that could be obtained from rinse samples taken during the pre-rinse and final rinse circuits of the CIP program. Pre-rinse samples were tested for the product specific assay to establish the challenge material concentration. Final rinse samples were tested using the same product specific assay to detect residual protein, pH and conductivity, to detect residual cleaning agents, and total organic carbon to detect any carbon containing residues which may have remained after cleaning.

SURFACE SAMPLING

A relatively recent addition to the sampling method portfolio for the biopharmaceutical industry is surface sampling. As a sampling technique, surface sampling is an effective means of directly evaluating the cleanliness of a production surface. Insoluble materials that may not have been removed during cleaning can be detected using a surface sampling technique such as swabbing. Surface sampling is commonly used in conjunction with or used to complement rinse water sampling to yield a complete cleaning picture.

Surface sampling by swabbing allows one to control the sampling area, thereby making the quantification of assay results easier (see Case Study 5.4) than for less direct sampling methods such as rinse water sampling. Sampling sites may include both accessible areas (tank walls) and hard to reach areas (valve diaphragms or gasket materials). Surface samples can be analyzed using a variety of testing methods including the following:

Surface Sampling Analytical Methods

• Total Microbial Count [see reference 2]

• Total Organic Carbon [3]

• Phosphate Residue [4]

• Last Component to Rinse (LCR) using HPLC [5]

Case Study 5.3

A formulation will be used to formulate multiple (3) concentrations of multiple (3) products. The solubility of the active ingredients and buffer components vary. Due to the possibility of cross contamination from potential product residues during formulation, the vali-

(Continued on page 111)

(Continued from page 110)
dation associated with this tank must focus on establishing evidence that the current cleaning procedures prevent this risk. A comprehensive testing scheme is developed which includes visual inspection, rinse water sampling, and surface sampling. The tank is cleaned per the established SOP and rinse samples are taken. The rinse samples are tested for the specific product that was in the tank previously, pH and conductivity, and total organic carbon. The tank is then disassembled, visually inspected, and (surface) sampled for total organic carbon. The validation testing is challenged with the most concentrated formulation batch for each product three times to prove that each product can be removed from the tank consistently. This strategy incorporates a worst case challenge for the product concentrations and is comprehensive in that all three products are used as challenge material.

Case Study 5.4

A surface sampling program is to be developed. A company currently produces two different proteins (Product A and Product B) formulated in the same tank. The cleaning validation program for this specific tank includes taking swab samples and testing for Total Organic Carbon. Using the results from the swabbing study the company wants to calculate the maximum theoretical amount of protein cross-contamination of Product A that could be present in a dose of Product B.

The process and sampling method variables that are used to equate the possible amount of cross-contaminating protein are outlined below followed by the actual calculations.

Surface Sampling Method

- Swab samples are taken using a Teflon® template with an interior surface area of 2" x 2".

- The swabs are then placed in a test tube containing 50ml of extraction solution.

- The limit of detection using this method was found to be 1 ppm.

Formulation Tank

- Interior product contact surface area = 2,365 in.^{2}

Product Information

- Percent carbon in Product A = 54.00%

(Continued on page 112)

(Continued from page 111)

- Standard dose of Product A = 0.3 mg/ml

- Formulation batch volume of Product B = 110 *l*

Assumptions

- A production formulation leaves contaminating residue on the formulation tank interior surface which is not removed or denatured by cleaning. The concentration of the remaining residue is 1 ppm.

- This assumes that all contaminating carbon detected is Product A.

- All of the contaminating Product A is uniformly distributed in the 110 *l* batch of Product B.

Calculations

EQUATION	NOTES
Step 1. Allowable Amount of Carbon Left on Equipment Surface per in^2	
1 ppm C = 1 mg C/*l*	C = Carbon
(1 mg C/1000 ml)(50 ml) = 0.05 mg C	1 ppm Carbon on swab is diluted into 50 ml of extraction solution.
0.05 mg C/4 in.^{2} = 0.0125 mg C/in.^{2}	Surface Area of sample is 4 in.^{2}
0.0125 mg C/in^2	This concentration represents the minimum amount of carbon that could be left on the tank walls and still be detected.
Step 2. Total Amount of Carbon	The total amount of carbon represents the amount of carbon left on the equipment surface per in.^{2} (Step 1) multiplied by the interior product contact surfacearea of the tank. This gives the totalamount of carbon that could be mixed into the next batch (the contaminating carbon concentration).
(0.0125 mg C/in.^{2})(2365 in.^{2}) = 29.56 mg C	
Step 3. Contaminating Carbon to Product A Conversion	The contaminating carbon concentration (Step 2) is converted to contaminating Product A concentration by multiplying by the ratio of carbon in Product A.
29.56 mg Carbon/54.00% Carbon in Product A = 54.74 mg Product A	
Step 4. Concentration of Contaminating Product A in a Product B Formulation	
54.74 mg (Product A)/110 *l* Product B = 0.5 mg (Product A)/*l* (Product B)	110 *l* is the Batch Size for Formulated Product B.
= 5.0 x 10^{-4} mg Product A/ml Product B	Convert units to mg/ml.

(Continued on page 113)

(Continued from page 112)

Step 5. Contaminating Dose of
Product A in a Dose of Product B.

(5.0 x 10⁻⁴ mg Product A/ml   0.3 mg/ml is the standard Product A
Product B)/(0.3 mg/ml Product A)   dose concentration

= 1.7 x 10⁻³ Doses of Product A
in 1 Dose Product B.

COUPONS

Cleaning effectiveness can be evaluated using coupons made from representative samples of materials of product contact surfaces. Typically, coupons are coated with an indicator soil and placed or hung inside production equipment during a cleaning cycle. The coupons are then removed and their surface a nalyzed for residues. Coupons simplify the surface sampling test procedures but are an indirect measure of the production surface cleanliness. Consequently, coupon sampling methods are often combined with other sampling methods such as rinse water data and visual inspection to create a total cleaning program.

SAMPLING METHOD RECOVERY

The use of surface sampling methods requires that an analysis be performed of the ability to recover the residue of interest from the surface being studied. Recovery studies are typically performed that correlate the sampling method to the surface and residue. Often, recovery studies use coupons with a known quantity of analyte/residue spiked onto the coupon surface. The surface is then analyzed using the surface analysis method of choice and the amount of material removed from the surface is correlated to the actual amount present. With this technique, recovery data can be established for a specific test procedure and performance qualification acceptance criteria adjusted accordingly.

Recovery studies can also be designed to better understand operator to operator variation in sampling technique. Under the controlled conditions of a recovery study, different operators can be used to determine the amount of inter-operator variance in sampling technique.

FACTORS IMPACTING SAMPLING PROGRAMS

Several important factors can affect sampling programs including operator training, sample stability and sample containers. Each of these factors should be considered when establishing a sampling program.

Training

One of the most important components of any sampling program is operator training. It is especially important that operators are completely trained in manual, frequently aseptic sampling practices. SOPs should be in place that explain how the sampling is to be performed and documentation attesting to each sampler's training. Consistency in sampling is the key to a successful study.

Sample Stability

Due to the high sensitivity of many of the analytical methods used to test cleaning validation samples, and the low concentrations of analytes, sample stability is an important consideration for a cleaning program. Often, an analyte will bind to the sample container or in some cases react with the solvent over time, thereby hindering subsequent analysis. Stability studies can be conducted to determine the ability to collect, store and re-use samples for a sampling program.

Sample Containers

As discussed above, not all containers are suitable for all sampling situations or they may need to be specially prepared (i.e., treated for TOC analysis). Assure that the container is not adversely effecting the recovery of the analyte by testing several container configurations/compositions. Clean containers are especially important for particulate analysis studies and for TOC samples, and should be tested for background levels of potential contaminants prior to selection.

A table comparing the various sampling methods and their advantages and disadvantages is provided on the next page.

SUMMARY

Many sampling techniques can be used to obtain cleaning validation data. Sampling techniques should be evaluated before use to determine what information can be gained by using each particular method. The evaluation should be based on the desired goals of the validation program, available analytical detection methods, the chemistry of the cleaning agents, and the physical geometry of the equipment. Once appropriate techniques are chosen sampling methods can then be used independently or in combination.

Table 5.1
Comparison of Sampling Methods

Sampling Method	Advantages	Disadvantages
Visual	Easy to do	Subjective
	Detects surface soils	All equipment not inspectable
	Points out worst case of contaminants	Doesn't detect low levels
	Minimal to no equipment required (good light source, mirror)	
Rinse Water Sampling	Easy to do; easy to collect samples	Doesn't detect adhering residues
	Detects soluble materials including cleaning agents	Large dilution effect making analyte recovery troublesome
	Can be used routinely to monitor progress of cleaning cycle	
Swabs	Detects adhering materials	Evaluation work (swab interference and recoveries) are time consuming
		Operator-to-operator variability
		Some equipment areas not accessible
		Entering or disassembling equipment may be required
Coupons	Can be removed from system for swabbing	Must be removed from system
	Conformational (piping elbows) and compositionally similar (316L SS)	Not representative of entire vessel

REFERENCES

1. Berry, I.A., Nash, R.A., "Cleaning Validation," *Pharmaceutical Process Validation*, Marcel Dekker, Inc., V57, 1993, pp 319–349.

2. Jenkins, K.M., Vanderwielen, A.J., "Cleaning Validation: An Overall Perspective," *Pharmaceutical Technology*, V18(4), April 1994, pp 60–73.

3. Strege, M.A., et al., "Total Protein analysis of Swab Samples for the Validation of Bioprocess Equipment," *Biopharm*, V7(9), November 1994, pp 40–42.

4. Garnick, R., et al., "a Total Organic Carbon Analysis Method for Validating Cleaning Between Products in Biopharmaceutical Manufacturing, *Journal of Parenteral Science and Technology*, V.45(1), January/February, 1991, pp 13–19.

5. Geigert, J., et al., "Role of Quality Control in Validation of Biopharmaceutical Processes: Case Example of Clean-in-Place (CIP) Procedure for a Bioreactor," *Journal of Parenteral Science and Technology*, V.48(5), September/October 1994, pp 236–240.

6

Analytical Methods That Support Cleaning Validation Studies

Methods that support cleaning validation studies may be either specific for a particular residue or non-specific in nature, detecting a wide variety of analytes. Examples of specific assays include immunoassays and chromatographic assays where a particular molecular species is detected. Specific assays are often used to document removal of a product prior to manufacturing changeover, removal of a specific detergent following initial cleaning, or to assay for an organic solvent which may have been present. These assays are often employed when the target analyte has unusual toxicity or antigenicity, during manufacturing changeover, or when only one protein is expected, e.g., during the last purification steps.

Examples of non-specific methods commonly employed include colorimetric protein determination, absorbance, pH, conductivity, and total organic carbon. These methods may indicate the presence of a wide variety of molecular species and are often valuable because of their broad specificity range.

The most common approaches to validation and monitoring of cleaning procedures have been analysis of rinse water, surface samples, and visual inspection.

In the first case, purified water is used as a final rinse of product contact surfaces. The rinse water is collected and both the source water and rinse water are tested. If the rinse water quality has degraded, it is assumed to be from residues on the surface which have rinsed off. Testing may include both specific and non-specific assays. In the past, testing was limited to USP test procedures for purified water. Today testing tends to be more robust and goes beyond the traditional USP test procedures. Only those residues which are soluble in the aqueous rinse are recoverable, hence residues in equipment areas which are inaccessible to rinsing may be underestimated. Other sections of this document deal with equipment design and sampling techniques related to these issues.

For those areas where rinse water analysis may not result in representative sampling, product contact surfaces may be swabbed and the residuals on the swab analyzed. The swab may be saturated with a solvent suitable for analyte removal and can be accurately related to a specific surface area. Validation of sampling techniques should demonstrate satisfactory recovery of expected residues for solvents employed as well as confirming solvent compatibility with the assay method. Depending on the assay to be employed, the residue may be removed from the swab and analyzed or the swab may be directly tested by combustion methods.

TYPES OF ANALYTES

Due to the nature of the biotechnology industry, many of the analytes which need to be tested during cleaning validation differ from those of the traditional pharmaceutical industry.

Proteins

The most obvious difference is the presence of large biomolecules, especially proteins. A major and easily defined analyte is residual final product, which is usually protein. However, unlike small molecules, the protein will potentially be present in several forms, complicating analysis. The forms include active protein, inactive but intact protein, and fragmented protein. Active final product may retain complete activity or may be only partially active. Intact but inactive final product may be denatured or simply rendered inactive by other physical changes such as chemical modification. Fragmented protein may be missing a single amino acid or may be in small pieces. Fragmentation can occur chemically or enzymatically. Particularly challenging to analysis is the uncertainty as to which of the forms will be present, as well as the heterogeneity of all forms. It is important to distinguish between analysis of proteins and analysis of cleaning agents in cleaning validation. A regulatory question in response to a license application by a biotechnology company stated:

> There should be an assay for each different product type. These assays are independent from those used to analyze the removal of cleaning agents [1].

In addition to proteins of known identity, biotechnology processes also leave other proteinaceous contaminants behind, including contaminating intracellular and extracellular proteins that are part of the starting host organism as well as proteins that are part of media components such as albumin. This class of analytes is very large and diverse; the types, sizes and characteristics are almost infinite. Thus, unlike final product, analysis of these proteins must necessarily be based on their identity as proteins and not related to any specific characteristic.

Organic Compounds

In addition to proteins, other cellular components can be left behind during a biotechnology production process. Since living organisms are the "factories" producing the biomolecules of interest, the types of contaminants potentially remaining after processing span the range of biomolecules found in nature, and their numbers are enormous. For example, *E. coli* is estimated to contain approximately 5,000 different kinds of molecules including some 3,000 proteins and 1,000 nucleic acids [2]. Potential residual biomolecules include: DNA, RNA, nucleotides, endotoxins, carbohydrates and lipids, as well as any fragments thereof.

The systems used to culture the living cells producing final product also have small organic molecule contaminants. For example a defined E. coli medium can contain glucose, lactose, amino acids, and vitamins; a mammalian medium can contain indicator dyes, insulin, transferrin and thimerisol.

Inorganic Compounds

The source of inorganic compounds in the production of biomolecules includes process components, medium components and cleaning solutions such as detergents and phosphates. During the process itself, buffers and salts are integral components of unit operations. Additionally, chaotropic agents and heavy metals may be part of the process. Salts present multiple problems for cleaning surfaces due to their corrosive nature; high viscosity chaotropic agents may also present unique problems. Several types of inorganic media components may be present in varying amounts, such as salts and phosphates. Cleaning solution inorganic molecules include phosphates, detergents, acids and bases.

Biological Contaminants

Biological residuals will vary greatly with the type of expression system. Airborne bacteria need to be considered in all types. Mammalian expression systems may include mycoplasma and viral contamination; bacterial expression systems may include viable and non-viable host bacteria in inappropriate places.

The presence of rich media in the early stages of a production process at room temperature or elevated temperature presents particular challenges for biological contaminants. Although these microbial contaminants are not present during the well controlled manufacturing process, they may sometimes be present following use and short term storage prior to sanitization and cleaning.

IN SITU VERSUS CENTRAL LABORATORY TESTS

Selection of an appropriate assay should include assessment of the assay's portability. Some analytical methods require minimal equipment, are quickly performed and need minimal data analysis. These techniques including pH, conductivity, and some types of TOC can be designed into process systems as in-line detectors. Other forms of these tests can use hand-held devices (e.g., conductivity meters, pH paper) which can be immediately applied during a procedure as initial indicators of cleanliness. Chromatographic testing, immunoassays and many other assays require more complex equipment and setup, data analysis procedures and, therefore, are usually confined to more centralized testing laboratories in most companies. For these reasons, both on-site and central testing are often performed during validation studies while subsequent routine monitoring of cleaning may use the simpler on-site procedures.

DETAILED METHOD EVALUATIONS

Different assays are appropriate for different applications. It is important to understand the assays, their capabilities and their limitations. Two general categories of assays can be identified based upon their specificity or lack thereof for a given residue. These categories are especially important for cleaning validation because of the need be able to test for a wide range of possible residues.

Residue Specific Assays

For residue specific assays, the analysis centers around a known compound, exploiting specific characteristics of that compound. In all residue specific assays, the assay is unique to the analyte. As this is a labor intensive process, it would be unusual to develop this assay solely for cleaning validation. Typically these assays are developed as part of QC analysis and process development and may have been used to define specifications. However, each method needs to be validated independently for each application. Validation of these assays for support of cleaning should include a thorough analysis of analyte response under cleaning conditions. Residue-specific assays are extremely important for product changeovers. One biotechnology company received several questions from the FDA regarding the mixture of different cell type products in their multiproduct facility, and the separation and cleaning validation related to their use [3].

The principle of Bioassays involves determining the specific activity of a molecule in an assay exploiting its biological activity. The bioassay can only be used for a molecule of known activity, typically (but not limited to) a final product. An advantage is that it is usually highly specific and can be highly sensitive; disadvantages include poor precision and detection of only those molecules that are active. Bioassays are an example of the unique activity(s) and detection methods of proteins relative to traditional pharmaceuticals. Although a biological product may not retain activity through rigorous cleaning procedures, bioassays can serve as valuable tools in cleaning validation.

Case Study 6.1

Company X produces a bacterial protein toxin for use in various vaccines. This protein is detoxified and purified during later steps in vaccine manufacturing. Fermentation and harvest equipment contact the bacterial toxin before detoxification. Because the fermentation and harvest equipment may contain raw bacterial toxin, the cleaning procedure for this equipment includes a heat inactivation (denaturation) step. Heat inactivation is followed by manual or clean-in-place (CIP) cleaning, depending on the equipment. Company X decided to validate the heat inactivation step separately from the remainder of the cleaning procedure. Company X's objective was to ensure that the heat inactivation procedure detoxified the protein before the equipment was disassembled for cleaning. Company X uses a cell culture based cytotoxicity assay to verify the detoxification of the protein. This assay was adapted and validated for use with the raw fermentor broth. Company X sampled 3 fermentation lots, both before and after the heat inactivation step. These samples were assayed for cytotoxicity using the cell culture assay. Results of the cell culture assay showed that the heat inactivation step detoxified the bacterial protein. Company X validated the remaining cleaning step using conventional assays such as Bradford protein and Total Organic Carbon.

Immunoassays are based on the recognition of an antigen by an antibody. There are many different types of assay configurations. The assay commonly involves a protein noncovalently bound to a solid phase (e.g., a microtiter plate), a protein in solution and a detection method [4]. The detection method is typically enzymatic (enzyme-linked immunosorbent assay, or ELISA) but can be based on other chemistries. The strength of immunoassays is their specificity, again exploiting the great diversity of proteins. Their weakness is somewhat poor reproducibility. The avidity of the antibody for the antigen and other issues influence the assay reproducibility; however, the assay can be quantitatively useful and several biotechnology companies use immunoassays in both cleaning validation and process monitoring. Typically, detection limits are in the range of 0.1–1 ng/ml. As with other specific assays, the validation of the assay application should include specificity studies using alternate forms such as denatured or aggregated protein and studies to identify any buffer or solvent effects on assay performance.

Another residue specific assay is high performance liquid chromatography (HPLC), although the method must be completely developed to be residue specific. Widely used in biotechnology [5], HPLC employs rigid microparticulate chromatographic matrices. The analytes that can be detected using this method include proteins, peptides and nucleic acids as well as small molecules. HPLC methods span different types of analytical chromatography including reverse phase, ion exchange, hydrophobic interaction, affinity chromatography and size exclusion. Once an assay has been developed, the specificity can be very high, although care needs to be taken to avoid co-elution of analyte and contaminants. HPLC methods can often distinguish chemical modifications of proteins, reduced vs. non reduced and unfolded vs. folded proteins. Accuracy and reproducibility are also very good with quantitative recoveries and 1–2% relative standard deviations common. Sensitivity can be good depending on the matrix; for example one study reported the minimal detectable amount of human growth hormone on RP-HPLC to be 0.7 µg [6]. Methods suitable for detection of nucleosides, nucleotides, polysaccharides, and detergents/surfactants are also available.

Another assay method unique to proteins is polyacrylamide gel electrophoresis (PAGE) [7]. This method separates proteins on the basis of molecular weight. It can be specific for a given protein (e.g., final product) or for a group of proteins (e.g., contaminating proteins). This method is widely used in the biotechnology industry in areas as diverse as fermentation tanks (early in the process) to formulation tanks (late in the process). The same assay would need to be validated and modified for the appropriate step in the process. The specificity is limited to proteins in the appropriate size range. Detection limits are typically 0.01-0.1 µg/band/lane for Coomassie-stained gels and 2–10 ng/band/lane for silver-stained gels (a non-linear but sensitive staining method). Colloidal Coomassie and gold stains may also be useful. Qualitative detection is highly reproducible, quantification is difficult but used in certain cases.

The main advantage of residue-specific assays lies in their specificity and the ability to detect known agents. This is particularly useful when cleaning validation needs to verify the removal (or quantify the presence) of known contaminants such as final product or process intermediates. These methods are especially useful during product changeover in a multiproduct facility.

Non-Specific Assays

In residue non-specific assays, analysis centers around the determination of various compound or component classes. The assay is not unique to the compound being analyzed and therefore can have broad application.

One of the most useful assay methods involves measurement of total organic carbon (TOC) present in a sample. With this technique, any organic carbon-containing molecule is detectable. Commercial organic carbon analyzers measure organic carbon after conversion to carbon dioxide. This involves some type of infra-red spectrophotometric detection and comparison to standards for quantification. TOC can be measured directly or can be determined as the difference between total carbon (TC) and total inorganic carbon (TIC).

Commercial instruments for automated TOC analysis use three primary methods for these measurements. High temperature combustion furnace instruments inject a sample into a combustion tube containing a chemical catalyst. The sample is heated to a high temperature, usually about 450°C in the presence of oxygen, converting the carbon present to CO_2. The CO_2 is then purged through a non-dispersive infrared (NDIR) detector and is quantified. This measurement defines the total carbon (TC) content of the sample. Another sample is then transferred to a secondary reactor where it is acidified, converting the inorganic carbon (IC) present to CO_2. The CO_2 is again purged into the NDIR detector and quantified. The IC is then subtracted from the TC to give a value for TOC. Many of these instruments also routinely measure non-purgeable organic carbon (NPOC) which is essentially equivalent to TOC in the absence of large concentrations of volatile organic species. For measurement of NPOC, the sample is first acidified and sparged to remove IC prior to injection into the high temperature catalyst tube.

Low temperature or UV-induced persulfate oxidation are the other major methods for TOC determination. In these instruments, a sample is injected into a reaction vial. Acid is added to convert the IC to CO_2 which is then purged from the sample and measured by NDIR. This same sample is then oxidized by addition of a persulfate solution while heated to 100°C or while exposed to UV light. The organic carbon is converted to CO_2 and measured by NDIR as a direct measurement of TOC.

A recent approach to TOC analysis uses UV/catalyst or UV/persulfate to generate the CO_2 but quantifies the CO_2 by direct conductivity or selective membrane conductivity.

A useful approach to validation of TOC for support of biopharmaceutical cleaning has been reported by Baffi, et al. [8]. Biological compounds including bovine serum albumin, sodium dodecyl sulfate, amino acids, dextrose, DNA, endotoxin, and several recombinant products were used to evaluate TOC with respect to sensitivity, linearity, limit of quantification, accuracy, precision, recovery and specificity toward denatured proteins. Using this approach, a TOC method can be validated with respect to its ability to detect any carbon-containing compound or to detect a specific residual product.

To assess residual protein in cleaning validation studies, several methods for estimating protein concentration are applicable. Most of these are colorimetric protein assays in which the concentration of protein is related to dye binding, which is determined spectrophotometrically [9]. Examples include the Biuret, Bradford, BCA and Lowry methods. The most commonly used of these is probably the Bradford method which measures Coomassie Brilliant Blue G-250 binding to protein. The dye binds non-covalently to basic or aromatic residues, causing the dye to shift from a red form to a blue form which is measured at 595 nM. All of these assays are simple, inexpensive and easily automated. The assays can detect protein concentrations at low µg/ml concentrations. Many of the assays are compatible with buffers, salts, detergents and other compounds often found in biopharmaceutical manufacturing systems. Since dye binding can vary considerably with different proteins, the reference protein should be validated against a typical protein residue when used in cleaning validation studies.

Case Study 6.2

Company X produces a recombinant protein on a very large scale. The protein becomes gelatinous upon denaturation and presents a challenge to surface sampling and quantitative techniques. A sampling method using polyester swabs and 5M NH_4OH as a solvent was developed which was validated to recover 60–98% of the protein depending on the denaturation state. Samples were analyzed for protein content using a BCA dye binding method in an automated microtiter plate mode suitable for analyzing the large number of samples generated. The quantitative limit of the assay was demonstrated to be 1.7 µg/ml.

Conductivity is a simple and effective method for measurement of residual ionic species. The conductivity/resistivity of dilute contaminants in rinse water is proportional to their concentrations. This method is especially appropriate for detecting acids, bases and salts at the ppm level. This method includes comparing the inlet and outlet resistivity of a CIP stream. For example, a 1 ppm of sodium hydroxide in pure water has a conductivity of 6 µS/cm and a similar concentration of phosphoric acid has a conductivity of 4 μS/cm. The operator must consider the pH and dissolved CO_2 content of the solution as both will affect conductivity measurements. Because of their zwitterionic nature and relatively low mobility, proteins are poor analytes for this method. Conductivity is, however, a very useful technique for detection of residual cleaning agents. Addition of conductivity to the Water for Injection (WFI) specifications in the USP is currently under consideration.

An additional non-specific and widely used measurement in cleaning validation is pH, primarily used for monitoring the removal of concentrated acids and bases used to clean residues from product contact surfaces. Several applications of pH measurements are commonly employed. These include use of pH paper, prepackaged solutions containing indicator dyes, and on-line and free standing potentiometric electrodes. It is important to remember that pH is a logarithmic expression of hydrogen ion concentration; therefore, a difference of 1 pH unit is indicative of a 10-fold difference in hydrogen ion content. pH measurements are among the simplest and most convenient methods to use in cleaning validation. Many of the process equipment components have built-in pH electrodes which can be utilized at fermentor and chromatographic sites. Use of pH in cleaning validation should be validated to demonstrate the effect on pH of expected excipients such as detergents, solvents, and salts. The effect of process stream temperature on pH must also be considered.

Some commonly used detergents are phosphate based. Many colorometric methods for residual phosphates are available. They generally involve use of various molybdate solutions and are sensitive to high ng levels of phosphate.

Absorbance (UV/VIS) scans of effluent streams can be used to detect specific absorbing compounds or can be used to monitor wavelengths which many biological compounds have in common. For example, nucleic acid and protein contaminants are maximally detectable at 254 and 278 nM respectively, and many cleaning agents and detergents also have specific absorption maxima which can be used to selectively monitor their presence.

A broad non-specific assay is total dissolved solids (TDS), which can be quantified as residual weight on drying. Total dissolved solids are usually expressed as a maximum allowable change in weight of a dish after having had 100 mL of water dried over a steam bath. Limits for WFI, for example, are 0.001%. Therefore, the contribution of solids due to product contact surfaces following a WFI rinse can readily be determined. This method, although useful, requires 5–6 hours for evaporation and is subject to a high number of false positives. It is thus of limited value in routine cleaning monitoring.

In analyzing rinse water, USP WFI tests can be used. These tests include several wet chemistry limit tests including those for the presence of chloride, carbon dioxide, calcium, heavy metals, oxidizable substances, total solids and pH. The tests are primarily visual colorimetric or turbidometric analyses which are non-quantitative in nature. Although many of the parameters measured are useful indicators of deterioration of WFI which may have been used as a final rinse of product contact surfaces, much more convenient, quantitative methods are available for most of the analytes. As a result, USP WFI tests are becoming less common in the industry.

A method that offers simultaneous analysis of several elements, very high sensitivities, reliable instrumentation and rapid analysis is inductively coupled plasma emission spectroscopy (ICP), a type of secondary emission spectroscopy utilizing stable high energy plasma excitation sources such as argon. The source of plasma is coupled in one of several ways to the sample and then injected into the spectrometer as an aerosol. The sample is excited by collision with high energy electrons and argon atoms and the light emitted is detected at wavelengths specific for each element. A typical analysis can simultaneously quantify 20–25 specific elements at ranges of 0.005–0.1 ppm in water. The method is, therefore, quite useful in detection and identification of buffer salts, leachates and other heavy metal contaminants present in cleaning studies.

METHODS COMPARISONS

In choosing the analytical methods for cleaning validation, it is important to choose the assay appropriate to the application and compatible with the sampling technique. For example, total organic carbon would be of little value when used with a carbon based swab; conductivity measurements would be quite useful following use of high salt concentrations for removal of residues.

The probability of developing a specific, sensitive assay for each analyte which might be encountered is not feasible in a biological production environment as products are produced in extremely complex cocktails often containing mammalian sera, protein growth promoting agents, mixtures of co-factors, vitamins, amino acids, salts, buffers, indicator dyes and complex cellular components resulting from the presence of the producing cell. Development of specific assays is extremely time consuming. Typically, assays with greater specificities require longer development time (see Figure 6.1).

It is often valuable, therefore, to select multiple methods for use in cleaning validation such that non-specific assays having high sensitivity and a broad specificity range are applied initially. If analytes are detectable with these assays, then one may proceed with more specific assay methods to identify which are the problematic species. Table 6.1 lists assays which are appropriate for different analytes. Some assays can be used for more than one analyte. TOC is becoming a widely used assay for many stages during a process. Additionally, different assays will be appropriate at different steps in the process. For example, product-specific assays are more appropriate for later steps, or in multiproduct facilities.

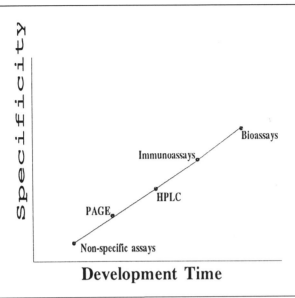

Figure 6.1
Higher Specificity Assays Require Longer Development Time

Table 6.1
Analyte to Assay Comparison

Type of Analyte	Assays
Protein	Bioassays, ELISA, HPLC, PAGE, protein determination assays, absorbance, TOC
Organic Compounds	TOC, absorbance, TDS
Inorganic Compounds	Conductivity, pH, orthophosphate, TDS, ICP
Biological Systems	Viable cell analysis

Careful choices of assay applications can lead to an efficient cleaning validation program.

SUMMARY

Methods available for support of cleaning validation include analyte specific and non-specific assays. None of these methods can serve as a stand-alone universal technique for demonstrating cleanliness of product contact surfaces. In practice, most manufacturers rely on the combination of these techniques most optimal for detection of the expected biological residues and cleaning reagents employed. A typical cleaning validation study might employ pH, conductivity, total organic carbon, detergent assays, and if a multi-product facility, a product-specific assay. Cleaning validation will often employ analysis of surface residuals while routine monitoring of cleaning following validation may rely more on rinse water analysis.

REFERENCES

1. Regulatory questions related to cleaning validation were made available to the PDA committee by several biotechnology companies for use in this document.

2. Lehninger, A.L., *Biochemistry*, Worth Publishers, New York, 1977.

3. FDA questions related to cleaning validation were made available to the PDA committee by several biotechnology companies for use in this documents.

4. *Methods in Enzymology, Immunochemical Techniques*, H. Van Vunakis and J.J. Langone, eds., Academic Press, San Diego, vol. 70, 1980.

5. *High Performance Liquid Chromatography in Biotechnology,* Hancock, W.S., ed., John Wiley and Sons, New York, 1990.

6. Christensen, T., Hansen, J.J., Sorensen, H.H., and Thomsen, J. in *High Performance Liquid Chromatography in Biotechnology,* Hancock, W.S., Ed., John Wiley and Sons, New York, 1990, pp 191–204.

7. *Electrophoresis,* 2nd Ed., A.T. Andrews, ed., Clarendon Press, Oxford, 1987.

8. Baffi, R., Dolch, G., Garnick, R., Huong, Y.F., Mar, b., Matsuhiro, D., Niepelt, b., Parra, C., and Stephan, M. *Journal of Parenteral Science and Technology* 45, 1991, pp 12–19.

9. Stofcheck, C.M., *Methods in Enzymology*, Vol. 182: M. Deutscher ed., Academic Press, San Diego, 1990, pp. 50–68.

7

Approaches to Establishing Cleaning Validation Acceptance Criteria

Biotechnology processes used to produce biopharmaceuticals differ from traditional biochemical or chemically synthesized pharmaceuticals and manufacturing methods. More specifically, biopharmaceuticals are usually large, complex molecules making characterization by analytical methods difficult. The biological activity of these proteins is dependent on maintenance of the molecular conformation. The biotechnology processes used to produce biopharmaceuticals involve significant sequential purification of the protein or polypeptide product in most cases. These fundamental differences in the properties and manufacturing methodologies between biopharmaceuticals and other drug substances and products create unique considerations for cleaning acceptability.

REGULATORY DIRECTION FOR ESTABLISHING CLEANING LIMITS

Guidance from the regulating agencies on the subject of cleaning acceptance criteria tends to be limited to generalized statements such as those found below:

> Equipment and utensils shall be cleaned to prevent contamination that would alter the safety, identity, strength, quality or purity of the drug product beyond the official or other set established requirements. [1]

> All surfaces that come in contact with products shall be clean and free of surface solids, leachable contaminants, and other materials that will hasten the deterioration of the product or otherwise render it less suitable for the intended use. [2]

This is the basic guidance given by the FDA for establishing the level of cleanliness of equipment and utensils used in the production of drug products. This requirement has been expanded into bulk drug substances, including products derived from the "new" biotechnology by the FDA with the statement:

> Residue limits established for each piece of apparatus should be *practical, achievable*, and *verifiable*. The manufacturer should be able to document, by means of data, that the residual level permitted is *scientifically sound*.[3–4]

The FDA has drawn the line on establishing more specific guidance with the statement:

> FDA does not intend to set acceptance specifications or methods for determining whether a cleaning process is validated. It is impractical for the FDA to do so due to the wide variation in equipment and products used throughout the bulk and finished dosage form industries [5].

ACCEPTANCE CRITERIA BASIS AND FACTORS

Practical, achievable and verifiable cleaning validation acceptance criteria for biotechnology processes are typically established using a combination of rational approaches and combining these with an analysis of one or more critical, process related factors.

Several rational approaches can be used to form the basis for determining the limits for cleaning acceptance criteria including:

- Process Clearance Capability
- Cleaning Capability
- Percentage of a Toxic Dose
- Percentage of Daily Dose
- Limits of Detection

Four critical factors that will impact and affect cleaning acceptance limits regardless of the approach are:

1. The manufacturing process

2. The product

3. The cleaning agent and the cleaning procedure

4. The sampling and analytical methods for residue detection

Approaches to integration of the basis for determining acceptance limits and the critical factors will be addressed in a step-wise approach. First, aspects of the different basis will be outlined. Then the progressive steps of the manufacturing process will be discussed and various bases for limit setting will be applied.

BASIS FOR ACCEPTANCE CRITERIA

Acceptance criteria can be based upon one or more of several different process criteria. These can be grouped loosely into two main categories, a process reduction capability category, and a dose related category.

For the dose related category, a common basis for limits includes percentages of toxic and daily doses. These approaches are more often applied in the latter stages of processing where potential contaminating residues are well known and characterized and consequently can be compared to known drug interaction data.

Within the process reduction capability category are several related but slightly different approaches including: process capability, cleaning capability, log reduction and limits of detection. Each of these approaches focuses on an analysis of what a given step or portion of a process is capable of doing—rather than looking at what the end effect of a limit has upon some later step in the process. While the limits derived using one of these techniques may appear less tangible than those of a dose related category, the use of statistical data can be used to strengthen the justification for such a limit.

Each of the different approaches is discussed in detail below.

Process Clearance Capability

This approach is based on the demonstrated capability of the purification process to clear or remove known impurities such as amino acids or process additives. During process development, clearance studies can be performed by challenging the purification process with spiked or known amounts of the challenge material. Such demonstrated process capability allows the establishment of limits for these impurities in fermentation/cell culture and recovery steps of typical biotechnology processes.

Cleaning Capability

Probably the most frequently used basis of establishing limits is to determine the actual effectiveness of the cleaning process to remove residual soils during normal operational conditions. In this case, limits are derived from samples taken during normal processing runs to determine what the "normal" level of residues is for a given unit operation. Assuming in-process product specification testing methods are in place to verify that the manufacturing process itself is performing effectively, this method can be used to establish reasonable acceptance limits for a process.

Statistical process control techniques are often applied when using cleaning process capability as the basis for establishing acceptance criteria or limits. In this case, upper and lower control limits can be established with confidence that if the cleaning process is operating within the control limits, then the cleaning process is in control and acceptable for use.

The use of cleaning capability data to establish acceptance limits is often tied to a dosage related residue analysis to verify that the control limits for a contaminant are acceptable from a dosage perspective.

Percentage of Toxic Dose

Acceptance limits can be based on dose based relationships. This approach applies a safety factor to established toxicity data for a possible contaminant. The safety factor is generally in the range of 0.01% to 10% of the toxicity and is usually used to set the limits for such materials as detergents, sanitizing agents and cross-contaminating proteins [6–7].

Application of dose based factors to the establishment of contaminant limits is most often applied in the last steps of the manufacturing process. This is because the latter steps of a manufacturing process will typically be the steps with the greatest chance of contaminating a final dosage form.

Percentage of Daily Dose

Like the previous approach, this approach again applies a safety factor but this time it is to the daily dose of a possible contaminant. Three factors considered when using daily dose as a basis are the level at which a product is normally considered to be non-active (usually taken as 10% of the normal dose), the safety factor and the robustness of the cleaning process. A percentage of 0.1%, 0.001 dose, has been used in the final formulation, fill and finish areas where the contaminant is another pharmaceutical product [see 6], [8–9].

Limits of Detection

Unfortunately, acceptance limits are often based upon the limit of detection for a given analytical method. Often this is done simply because it is easy and fast. However, as with most such solutions, there are drawbacks. In this case, the drawback is that as analytical methods improve, the limits of detection will increase resulting in potentially unreasonable future acceptance limits. Regardless, use of the analytical limit of detection is frequently employed for the determination of cleaning acceptance limits.

FACTORS SUPPORTING CLEANING ACCEPTANCE LIMITS

Regardless of the approach taken to establish acceptance criteria, several critical factors must be considered. These factors will impact the ability to establish reasonable and achievable limits for a process or step in a process. Two of the factors, the manufacturing process and the product will most certainly impact the establishment of any related cleaning limit criteria and are discussed in detail below.

Manufacturing Process

Most biotechnology processes have distinct steps grouped as upstream and downstream processing. The establishment of cleaning limits for bioprocessing applications will often be dependent on the position of the step in the overall process. This is due in part to the "self-cleaning" nature of most biotechnology based purification processes, and is also due to the different nature of the residues themselves at each step of the manufacturing process.

Typically, cleaning acceptance criteria become more stringent the further downstream in the process the step is. This generalization is based upon the increased risk of contamination of an actual product dosage form the closer one gets to the final manufacturing process step.

Each step should be examined and then analyzed as part of the overall process to establish a reasonable and achievable acceptance limit.

Fermentation/Cell Culture

Fermentation/cell culture is a step during which cell growth occurs and product (or product precursors) are produced in the living host organism. The major emphasis on the cleanliness for this step is the elimination of any contaminant that will be carried through the isolation and purification steps to the final bulk substance. Potential product residuals following cleaning at this stage of the bioprocess include a wide range of cellular components such as proteins, polypeptide chain fragments, nucleic acids, carbohydrates and endotoxins in addition to the pharmaceutical active drug substance. The potential effect of such contaminants on subsequent fermentation or cell culture could include altering reproduction and growth, either of the same product or other products. This requires adequate cleaning to insure producing the desired protein. The longer and more complex the purification process, the more likely that such contaminating substances would be eliminated. Therefore, the concerns for cumulative residual build-up throughout in the expansion and product formation are of less concern.

Isolation

Harvesting of the cells or cell products is the first crude purification step where the product is separated from a large number of materials that are widely divergent from the product. This is often accomplished by centrifugation, filtration, capture chromatography or some combination of each. The isolation steps are early in the purification process and consequently will typically have a higher acceptance limit for cleaning if it is known that the possible contaminants will be removed in the downstream purification process. For example, cleaning acceptance criteria for a centrifuge used to concentrate cell solids may be 5–10 times higher than those for final purification equipment.

Initial Purification

More complex processes can require several purification steps after isolation of the product or precursor. Steps up to a renaturation in which the final active product is formed may be considered to be in this category and may entail chromatography, membrane separations, and other filtration. These methods are highly selective for the product and are designed to remove impurities of similar chemical functionality and physical properties to the desired product [10]. Levels of contaminants in the initial purification become more of a concern than during fermentation processes. Subsequent steps may not be designed to remove the impurities formed in these types of processes or may cause degradation products that will not be removed. Again, in the initial purification steps, the range of impurities can be significant so assays that can measure a broad spectrum of protein products should be used.

Final Purification

Final purification typically is indicative of an active product in the last steps of purification of the final bulk drug substance. This may include a series of chromatographic steps, filtration and drying. The purity in these steps is usually in excess of 95% and frequently above 99%. The levels of impurities allowed in these steps usually must be below the drug product published specification limits for foreign proteins such as host cell proteins, microbial content, related substances and other substances used in the processing. These established limits are the limits set in the Product License Application/New Drug Application or such standards as the United States Pharmacopoeia (USP). The impurities must be identified and quantified especially if there is the possibility of cross contamination from one product to another. Several approaches to quantifying the acceptable level of contamination are given in the next section on final formulation.

Final Formulation

In the final formulation steps, the bulk drug substance is converted to the final drug product by a series of steps that may include sterile filtration, formulation, filling and possibly freeze drying to produce the final dosage form. These operations do not usually include further purification. The cleaning procedure must therefore prevent the possibility of impurities being introduced above an established acceptable level. Since the number and types of impurities in these steps is usually due to cross contamination from another product that was previously processed in the equipment, identification and acceptable levels can be determined. A method for calculating cleaning validation acceptance limits for the final stages of processing has been presented by Mullen and Forman [9].

In summary, most of the official or other set established product purity limits address the level of contamination in the final drug product. Translating this into cleaning acceptance criteria for the earlier steps of the bioprocesses used in the production of the bulk biopharmaceutical substances requires evaluating the validity of setting a limit on contaminants that are known to be removed in subsequent processing steps. When dealing with proteins produced in microbiological hosts or cell cultures, a few unique aspects must be remembered. First, the contaminants from the hosts are complex and may not be well characterized. Second, all proteins behave differently. This may prevent the use of reference proteins to demonstrate the capabilities of cleaning techniques.

Acceptance criteria for steps in the upstream stages of the manufacturing process (seed culturing, fermentation, initial purification) should be workable from the process perspective. That is, because of the downstream purification steps, it is often more of a concern to ensure consistent operation of the equipment by preventing excessive product or by-product accumulation. On the other hand, acceptance criteria for the downstream steps of the manufacturing process (final purification, final bulk, filling); need to reflect acceptable residues per dosage of final product.

Use of Cleaning System Capability to Set Acceptance Limits

The design of clean-in-place (CIP) systems may produce better cleaning in the front-end of the process than the required limits. This can be depicted by the following generalized chart (see Figure 7.1).

The consideration for setting an acceptance limit then is to have limits which indicate the acceptable operation of the CIP equipment. Meeting this criteria will always insure that the impurity level is well below the acceptable range.

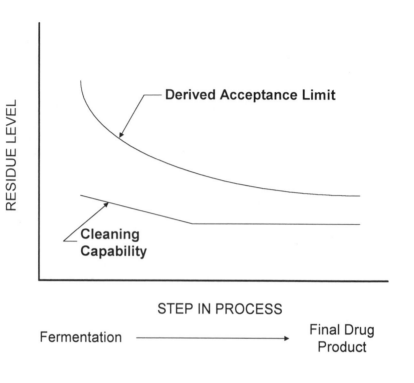

Figure 7.1
Cleaning System Capability and Acceptance Limits

Case Study 7.1: Use of Cleaning System Capability and Process to Set Acceptance Limits

Company ABC installed a CIP system to clean their fermenters and isolation equipment. The 10-minute CIP cycle for the 5,000-liter fermenter produced rinse water cleaning results that consistently demonstrated the ability to remove non-specific protein below 50 ppm as measured by a Total Organic Carbon (TOC) analysis. Additionally, after the CIP cycle, there was no visual evidence of product or detergent residual.

(Continued on page 137)

(Continued from page 136)

Smaller-scale, pre-production cleaning studies had demonstrated that residual non-specific protein was reduced to less than 100 ppm when hand washing procedures were used and still yielded acceptable product as determined by product specific assays.

Based on the bench scale studies that demonstrated that at 100 ppm, there was no impact on product quality, and the baseline data obtained from the operational CIP system, 50 ppm was established as the acceptance criteria for all equipment prior to the final bulk stage.

The Product

When establishing acceptance criteria for cleaning processes, it is often the product itself that is of most interest. This is especially true for multi-use facilities where carry-over or cross-contamination from one product to the next is one of the primary concerns. Even in single use or dedicated facilities, it is often the product or product intermediates that are being sampled for and consequently must have reasonable acceptance criteria established.

Concern for product residue carryover is most often associated with the final stages of processing where there is little chance of the process itself having the ability to clear or reduce any remaining product residue from the process stream. At this stage in the manufacturing process, dose based criteria are often considered. For products that are immunogenic or toxic at very low concentrations, e.g., some enzymes, vaccines and prostaglandins, the minimal reactive quantity per sample size should be determined and a medical "margin of safety" added for the acceptance criteria.

Once a reasonable residue limit has been determined, based for example on a dosage factor, then one can work backwards to establish reasonable acceptance criteria for the specific step in the process. (See Chapter 5: Sampling Methods, Case Study 5.4)

The establishment of reasonable acceptance criteria requires the judicious use of reasonable assumptions. Often, many different assumptions must be made in cleaning validation studies. Each should be evaluated and compared against known data to verify the validity of the assumption. Several common cleaning assumptions include:

- Uniform residue distribution on surfaces

- Uniform residue distribution within rinse solvent batch

- Uniform dispersement of contaminant residue in next batch

Acknowledgment should be made that a given assumption may be valid for one step in a manufacturing process and invalid in a different step of the same process. In some cases for example, the dissolution of a powder contaminant within a liquid is problematic, making the assumption of uniform residue distribution within the rinse solvent questionable.

Case Study 7.2: Use of Product Daily Dose to Set Acceptance Limits

Company ABC manufactures product XYZase, a highly reactive enzyme produced extracellularly by genetically engineered *E. coli*. Currently, XYZase is the only product licensed and produced in their facility. The therapeutic dose of XYZase is 10mg intravenously. It was demonstrated during product development that a 10μg dose of XYZase is non-reactive and there are no known allergic responses to XYZase. Therefore, ABC determined that 1/1,000 of the final dose of the specific protein would be their acceptance criteria for swabs taken from surfaces of cleaned final bulk tanks and filling equipment.

Case Study 7.3: Use of a Safety Factor to Set Acceptance Limits

The ABC Product Development group is ready to scale up the manufacturing process of a new product, DEFase, also an enzyme produced extracellularly by genetically engineered *E. coli*. DEFase is a toxic protein that has a potential killing mechanism against some tumors. The minimum therapeutic dose for DEFase has been shown to be 1 mg. The ABC Quality Control group has demonstrated that the TOC analysis measures a broad range of impurities (including denatured proteins) in the 0.1–10 ppm range. Product Development has shown that DEFase is non-reactive at 10 ppm, and that small scale fermenters, tanks, etc. could be cleaned to a less than 1 ppm range using a lengthened caustic wash cycle.

To bring the new product into the licensed facility/equipment, ABC wrote a cleaning validation protocol that included a modified CIP cycle (similar to the smaller scale process) with a TOC acceptance criteria of ≤1 ppm. (non-reactive level + 1 log safety factor) They then began compiling a validation database generated concurrently with clinical production batches of DEFase.

The point of these examples is that the development of cleaning validation, including acceptance criteria, needs to begin during the product development cycle. A thorough understanding of the process (both manufacturing and cleaning), the cleanability of the relative pieces of manufacturing equipment, and the impact of product residues are essential to setting reasonable limits.

The preferred approach to any validation study is a prospective one. That is, one should design the experiment including hypotheses, methods and acceptance criteria prior to the initiation of the study. Unfortunately, in the "real world" of cleaning validation, this is not always possible for full-scale manufacturing processes. It is not unusual for initial batches of product in large fermenters or chromatography systems to be clinical batches or even qualification/validation lots, (potentially) destined for market. Therefore, a concurrent validation approach to cleaning must often be followed.

To successfully complete a concurrent validation study, sufficient "development scale" data and a well characterized process are necessary to be able to set reasonable and scientifically sound cleaning validation acceptance criteria. In the examples, company ABC needs to know both products, XYZase and DEFase, and their respective cleanability, and must completely understand the manufacturing processes to establish meaningful cleaning validation acceptance criteria, prior to manufacturing DEFase clinical lots.

The Cleaning Agent and Cleaning Procedures

Many cleaning agents used to clean pharmaceutical manufacturing equipment may leave residues that may be considered a contaminant. These cleaning agents are usually ionic salts and may also contain surfactants. At the dilution of use, these are generally innocuous. Most assays for these organic residues are accurate in the 10–100 ppm range.

As has been discussed in previous sections of this document (see Chapters 3 and 4), typical CIP cycles include a caustic cycle, an acid cycle and multiple rinses with purified water and/or water for injection. Many cleaning detergent solutions are excellent solvents for removing proteins. However, these chemicals can also be very corrosive to stainless steel.

Case Study 7.4: Use of Visual Detection to Set Acceptance Limits

Company ABC installed a CIP system for its fermenters used to manufacture XYZase. The chemistry analytical department in conjunction with the process development scientists determined that a 1 N NaOH solution easily denatured XYZase, and residual product was effectively removed from the manufacturing equipment surfaces. The CIP cycle was consequently developed using 1N NaOH and a purified water rinse. The lab developed and validated a swab sampling procedure in conjunction with their analytical method and demonstrated a consistent 75 ppm residual Na level. That level of cleaning agent residue was shown to not adversely affect the product. So the acceptance criterion was set at < 100 ppm. After one year of manu-

(Continued on page 140)

(Continued from page 139)
facturing XYZase, the manufacturing operators noticed a discoloration on the inside surfaces of the fermenters. The material was scraped off of the stainless steel surface and the resultant analysis revealed iron compounds, typical of corroded stainless steel. Intensive acid treatment removed the discoloration.

The routine CIP cycle was modified to include a mild acid rinse after the purified water post-caustic rinse. This additional step and a final purified water rinse neutralized and more effectively removed the caustic detergent to levels around 10–25 ppm, and the discoloration on the inside of the fermenters did not reappear.

This example is hypothetical and the fictitious numbers are relevant only to ABC's cleaning agent sampling method and cleaning procedures. However, the example demonstrates that one must be concerned with not only the effect of the cleaning procedure and cleaning agents on residual product, but also on the processing equipment.

The Sampling Method and Analytical Methods for Residue Detection

A number of different analyses have been discussed (see Chapter 6). Technology has advanced methodology and analytical equipment to be able to detect very low concentrations of generic protein, specific protein, endotoxin, cleaning agent residue, etc. Of course, all sampling techniques and subsequent analyses should be validated to demonstrate an acceptable recoverability, precision and reproducibililty. Good scientific rationale should be applied to the establishment of reasonable acceptance criteria.

Case Study 7.5: Acceptance Criteria Based Upon Analytical Method Sensitivity

Company ABC has demonstrated that the XYZase process and product requires that their filling equipment be cleaned to less than 1/1,000 of the product final dosage form. However, the lab demonstrated that the analytical assay is capable of detecting nanogram quantities of the specific protein, which correlates to 1/1,000,000 of a final dosage form. In order to attain that level of cleaning of ABC's filling equipment, the equipment had to be extensively cleaned with detergents, ultrasonic cleaners, and lengthy hot Water for Injection (WFI) rinses. Consequently the total cleaning cycle took excessive time and materials. Analytical capabilities must be considered when

(Continued on page 141)

(Continued from page 140)
establishing acceptance criteria. However, the requirements of the product, the manufacturing process and the cleaning process must all be factored into the acceptance criteria rationale.

SUMMARY

In summary, the approach to establishing acceptance criteria to validate cleaning processes should include the following:

1. Knowledge of the product and process
   * How toxic or reactive is the product?
   * Is the process cumulative or are the steps to reduce residuals inherent in the process?
   * What is a medical margin of safety for the residual product on the subsequent product in the same equipment?

2. Knowledge of the cleaning agent and cleaning process
   * How rinsable is the detergent?
   * What impact does the residual detergent have on subsequent product?

3. Knowledge of the analysis used to detect residuals after cleaning
   * Are the methods validated within the determined sensitivity range (margin of safety?)
   * Is the limit of detection a reasonable limit for the cleaning process?

With this knowledge, the basis for establishing the criteria that best demonstrates the cleaning system capability and insures that subsequent products will not be contaminated can be selected. The testing which defines validation will then have a definitive demonstration of practical, achievable and verifiable limits.

REFERENCES

1. Food and Drug Administration, *Current Good Manufacturing Practice for Finished Pharmaceuticals*, April 1, 1987.

2. Code of Federal Regulations, Title 21, Part 600, para 600.11(b) U.S. Government Printing Office, Washington, D.C., revised April 1, 1991.

3. Food and Drug Administration, *Guide to Inspection of Bulk Pharmaceutical Chemicals,* U.S. government Printing Office, Washington, D.C., September 1991.

4. Food and Drug Administration, *Biotechnology Inspection Guide,* U.S. Government Printing Office, Washington, D.C., November 1991.

5. Food and Drug Administration, *Guide to Inspection of Validation of Cleaning Processes*, U.S. government Printing Office, Washington, D.C., July 1993.

6. Agalloco, J., "Points to Consider in the Validation of Equipment Cleaning Procedures," *Journal of Parenteral Science and Technology*, 46(5), 1992, pp 163–168.

7. Bader, F.G., Bum, A., Garfinkle, B.D., MacFarland, D., Massa, T., Copmann, T.L., "Multiuse Manufacturing Facilities for Biologicals," *Biopharmaceuticals*, 5(7), 1992, pp 34–42.

8. Fourman, G.L., Mullen, M.V., "Determining Cleaning Validation Acceptance Limits for Pharmaceutical Manufacturing Operations," *Pharmaceutical Technology*, 17(4), 1993, pp 54–60.

9. Jenkins, K.M., Vanderwielen, A.J., "Cleaning validation: An Overall Perspective," *Pharmaceutical Technology,* 18(4), 1994, pp 60–73.

10. Better, P.A., Cussler, E.L., Hu, W., *Bioseparations, Downstream Processing for Biotechnology*, John Wiley & Sons, New York, 1988.

Section III

MULTIPRODUCT CONCEPTS

Section I established the design concepts necessary to develop cleanable equipment and cleaning systems. Section II covered the validation process and the corresponding concepts including sampling methods, assay methodologies associated with cleaning validation, and acceptance criteria.

Section III discusses the concepts associated with multiproduct manufacturing. **Chapter 8** carefully examines the need for multiproduct manufacturing technoloy covering the economic and practical realities facing today's biotechnology companies. The concept of Changeover as it relates to multiproduct facilities and the advantages of dedicated versus non-dedicated equipment is also explored to provide the reader with a foundation for designing a sound multiproduct manufacturing program. All aspects of equipment use in a multiproduct facility are covered, including processing equipment, cleaning equipment, and the handling and preparation of raw materials.

The information contained in Section III provides the reader with an overview of the techniques and technologies used in today's multiproduct manufacturing facilities and the rationale that can be used to establish a practical changeover program.

8

Special Issues for Multiproduct Facilities

The topic of cleaning validation in multiproduct biotechnology facilities is becoming increasingly important as more biotechnology companies bring their first products to market. The FDA has made it clear, via seminars, articles, and 483 observations, that a sound cleaning validation program is essential for the approval of multiproduct biotechnology facilities [1].

Many biotechnology companies do not understand the magnitude or importance of cleaning validation in a multiproduct facility until the first pre-approval inspection nears. At this time, the pressure to come up with a program is intense. However, if this intensity is not tempered with foresight, the resulting program may not be easily applicable to future products. As a result, care must be taken when developing the program to ensure that it is not only rational, but that it can be reasonably applied to subsequent products. If time is not taken to ensure that the initial approach developed for the first product can be used for subsequent products, a great deal of resources will be expended for each new product.

This section will address those items that differ between multiproduct and dedicated facilities as they relate to the development of a cleaning validation program. Specifically, this section will discuss the need for multiproduct facilities, the changeover program, and equipment considerations.

THE NEED FOR MULTIPRODUCT FACILITIES

The need for multiproduct biotechnology production facilities arises largely from the desire of manufacturers to minimize the cost, risks, and time associated with bringing new products to market [2]. The initial investment in biotechnology production facilities is costly because of the many special features that are typically required. Building a facility, then, means that a large capital expenditure must be made, usually before the efficacy of the product has been fully demonstrated. This investment decision must be made early in the product's development since it is not uncommon for the late phase clinical trial material to be made in the initially licensed facility. The typical time frame (see Figure 8.1) and uncertainties associated with realizing a return on this investment mean that embarking on the construction of a facility is risky, especially for most young, cash poor biotechnology companies. These costs and risks are part of doing business in the industry; however, they can be reduced substantially by the use of multiproduct facilities.

With increasing pressure to control health care costs, minimizing the cost of biotechnology production facilities, and therefore the ultimate cost to produce the products of biotechnology, is essential and good business sense. However, biotechnology products, like all pharmaceuticals, are subject to the Code of Federal Regulations, and as a result, must be produced under CGMP conditions in licensed facilities [4–5]. These requirements on processing and facilities are by their nature very costly.

The costs are largely due to the following typical components of a biotechnology manufacturing facility:

1. Specialized utilities (water systems, HVAC, cold rooms) and process piping [6]

2. Adequate floor space for proper personnel and equipment flow patterns [see 1]

3. Specialized equipment and surface finishes

4. A comprehensive environmental monitoring program

These typical facility attributes have evolved as a result of the inherent aspects of most biotechnology products—they are typically heterogeneous, are often heat labile, and are subject to microbial contamination [7].

One may be able to argue the need for some or all of the above facility requirements, but there is no argument that they are costly. Several sources estimate the cost of typical biotechnology manufacturing floor space at anywhere from $200–$1,600 per square foot [3, 7–10]. If a company chooses to build a dedicated facility for each product entering late phase clinical testing, multiple large capital expenditures are necessary. One way to reduce the need

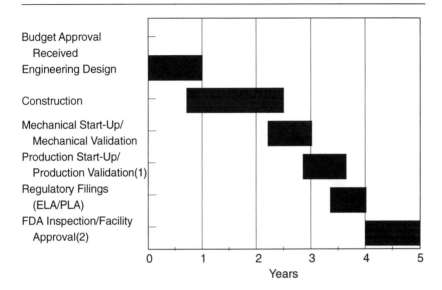

Budget Approval
  Received
Engineering Design

Construction

Mechanical Start-Up/
  Mechanical Validation
Production Start-Up/
  Production Validation(1)
Regulatory Filings
  (ELA/PLA)
FDA Inspection/Facility
  Approval(2)

0   1   2   3   4   5
Years

1. Assumes generation of consistency batches *prior* to filing.
2. Assumes success of the user fee program. Previously, time frames have
   been much longer.

Figure 8.1
Typical Facility Approval Cycle

for multiple expenditures is to build facilities which are designed to manufacture multiple products.

A multiproduct facility is a facility that is designed to accommodate the production of two or more products concurrently or on a campaigned basis. In a multiproduct facility designed solely for concurrent manufacturing, capital efficiency is achieved through the use of centralized utilities [11] and support services (warehouse, QC labs). In the case of a multiproduct facility designed solely for campaigned manufacturing, capital efficiency is achieved by eliminating the need for large expenditures for manufacturing equipment and floor space for each new product. Multiproduct facilities that are designed for both concurrent and campaigned manufacturing achieve capital efficiency in both ways. Therefore, multiproduct facilities can be an important element in the effort to control pharmaceutical, and therefore, health care costs.

Multiproduct facilities can also reduce the financial risk associated with bringing a new product to market. The primary risks associated with products at the development stage are that the product will never make it to the market and that the actual market for the product will be too small to return the investment needed to develop it. The use of a multiproduct facility can minimize these risks because a multiproduct facility allows a biotechnology company to advance several products using one facility. As a result, the initial capital investment in the facility can be spread over several potential products. If one or more of the products does not make it to market, then the investment in the facility can be carried by the other product(s). Furthermore, the ability to spread the expenditure over several product candidates may make a substantial difference in the effective cost of the drug, especially for a small indication product. Therefore, the ability to use a multiproduct production facility may make the difference in whether or not a company pursues a small indication product.

Finally, multiproduct biotechnology manufacturing facilities can reduce the time it takes to bring a product to market. As depicted above in Figure 8.1, the typical time frame from conceptual design to facility licensure is 5–7 years. With a multiproduct facility, time can be saved because the conceptual design, construction, equipment purchase, mechanical start-up, and mechanical validation steps do not have to be repeated for each new product. In addition, facility regulatory filings prepared for the first product can substantially reduce the amount of work needed to prepare them for the second and subsequent products. Therefore, multiproduct facilities can potentially save time in the typical product licensure scenario.

In conclusion, multiproduct facilities are an important element in the struggle to keep health care costs down. Multiproduct facilities can also reduce the risk and time associated with bringing a new product to market. These savings are especially important to biotechnology companies, who are typically young and cash poor.

THE CHANGEOVER PROGRAM

Changeover is unique to multiproduct facilities. Several activities are generally encompassed by the term changeover, one of which is cleaning non-dedicated equipment. A typical changeover sequence might encompass the following tasks:

- Remove any remaining prior product batches and samples

- Discard any disposable equipment or supplies

- Clean and store dedicated equipment

- Clean non-dedicated equipment

- Clean and sanitize production area surfaces (e.g., walls, floors, counters)

- QA review and release of production area for next product

It is the fourth task that is the subject of this section of the book. As alluded to earlier, the FDA has made it clear that cleaning procedures used on non-dedicated equipment during changeover must provide assurance that non-dedicated equipment has been cleaned sufficiently so as not to alter the safety, identity, strength, quality, or purity of the next product to be produced. There are several ways one can prove the success of cleaning procedures. One could test the cleaned equipment for the absence of product and/or appropriate contaminants following each cleaning. This method will be referred to in this chapter as verification. One could also conduct a prospective series of tests following cycles of use and cleaning. This method will be referred to in this chapter as validation. One could also start out by testing following each cleaning procedure until enough repeats of the procedure have been executed to validate the cleaning procedure. This method will be referred to in this chapter as the combination approach.

Verification of changeover includes appropriate sampling and testing at every changeover to ensure that non-dedicated equipment has been properly cleaned. Following the successful completion of the appropriate tests, the non-dedicated equipment is released for use with the next product. The verification approach is typically used when the planned number of changeovers is low, the test conditions are difficult to generate, or the test conditions are variable. The verification method has the advantage of saving time initially because the data collection and analysis are conducted concurrently with changeover. However, this method requires a higher level of effort over a longer period of time because the assay work will occur intermittently.

An example of how the verification approach to changeover might be applied is as follows:

Case Study 8.1

Company ABC uses a continuous fermentation process in the production of two different products, W and X. Both of these products are produced in the same non-dedicated processing equipment, on a campaigned basis. Current market demand for these products can be met by producing W for three months per year and by producing X for six months per year. Therefore, a changeover from W to X will occur approximately once per year, and a changeover from X to W will also occur approximately once per year.

Let us focus on changeovers from W to X. Since the W production process is continuous, some equipment, such as the fermentor, might only be cleaned after producing W once per year. Therefore, there would be only one opportunity per year to test the ability of the cleaning procedure to remove W from the fermentor. In addition, the "dirty" condition of the fermentor at the end of the

W production campaign would be tough to simulate for validation purposes, since the actual production process uses the fermentor continuously for three months at a time.

As a result of the above two factors, the infrequency of changeovers and the difficulty of generating the "dirty" condition, the verification approach to changeover might be used. Using this approach would mean that following the completion of each production campaign (for W and X), the non-dedicated equipment would be cleaned, and a full battery of testing would be conducted to ensure that the equipment is fit for use in the next production campaign.

A second approach to changeover that can be taken is a prospective validation of the changeover cleaning procedures. In this approach, the changeover cleaning procedures are tested multiple times (i.e., validated) to ensure that they clean the non-dedicated equipment adequately. This approach is typically chosen when the planned frequency of changeovers is high and/or the test conditions are relatively easy to generate for validation purposes. This approach has the advantage of allowing an organization to conduct the majority of the assay work in one large effort. However, this approach requires time up front to show repetition of the procedures. Once the changeover procedures are validated, the testing done at each changeover can be greatly reduced or eliminated.

An example of how the validation approach to changeover might be applied is as follows:

Case Study 8.2

Company DEF uses a batch cell culture process in the production of its two products, Y and Z. Both of these products are produced in the same non-dedicated fermentation equipment, on a campaigned basis. The fermentation processes take less time than the purification processes, so it makes sense economically to have one fermentor supplying two different purification trains. The optimal production scheme has been determined to be alternating the production of Y and Z in the fermentor on a weekly basis. Therefore, a changeover from Y to Z will occur approximately every two weeks, and a changeover from Z to Y will also occur approximately every two weeks.

Let us focus on changeovers from Y to Z. Since the Y production process will be run for one week and then the equipment will be changed over to produce Z, a relatively short period of time is necessary to get multiple tests of the cleaning procedure to remove both Y and Z. In addition, the "dirty" condition of the fermentor would be easier to generate for validation purposes, since the maximum length of any one run is only one week.

As a result of the above two factors, the frequency of changeovers and the relative ease of generating the "dirty" condition, the validation approach to changeover might be used. Using this approach would mean that the full battery of tests need only be performed until the reproducibility of the cleaning procedures to remove both products Y and Z could be demonstrated.

A third approach to changeover that can be taken is a combination of the verification and validation approaches. In this concurrent approach, the initial changeover periods are treated using the verification method, sampling and testing at each changeover. Successful completion of the appropriate tests would release the non-dedicated equipment for use with the next product. The verification approach is then continued until multiple changeovers have demonstrated that the changeover cleaning procedures perform in a consistent manner. When the goal of demonstrating consistency has been met, the changeover procedures can be considered validated, and the testing done at each changeover can be greatly reduced or eliminated.

An example of how the combination approach to changeover might be applied is as follows:

Case Study 8.3

Company ABC, described above, is successful in its production of products W and X using the same non-dedicated processing equipment. Three years pass since the start of production in the W and X manufacturing facility. During these three years, there have been three changeovers from W to X and three changeovers from X to W, using the same changeover cleaning procedures each time. In all, six sets of changeover data have been collected.

During all six changeovers, the appropriate sampling and testing indicated that the changeover cleaning procedures were effective in preparing the non-dedicated equipment for the production of the next product. As a result of the multiple successful changeovers, the changeover cleaning procedures can now be considered validated, and the testing done at each changeover can be greatly reduced or eliminated.

A recent question that many companies are struggling with is exactly what testing is required at changeover when the changeover procedures are validated. Intuitively, if one is able to validate changeover procedures using multiple representative studies, there should be no need for additional testing during changeover. However, recent indications are that the FDA does not share the same philosophy. At a roundtable session at the March 1992 PDA meeting, one industry representative stated that during a recent inspection, the FDA indicated that it wants to see some degree of testing at every changeover, regardless of whether the changeover procedures are validated. As a result of these recent trends, it is important that companies understand that, in a multiproduct facility, the cleaning validation program is an ongoing effort.

This ongoing effort is needed not only to design and execute validation studies, but also to allow constant attention to industry trends.

As alluded to in the introduction, the development of the changeover program should be done in a manner such that all of a company's current and future products can be covered. If the initial program lacks this flexibility, significant resource expenditures will be required to adapt the program to fit each new product.

Case Study 8.4

It is quite conceivable that one company might be producing all four of the products described above (W, X, Y, and Z). Let us assume that this company (GHI) develops and produces W and X first. At this time, Company GHI decides to use the verification approach to changeover, and it sets this approach forth in various official documents—SOPs, Validation Master Plans, etc.

Then, several years later, products Y and Z come out of development and into manufacturing. Company GHI now has a dilemma to face. If it proceeds to use the verification approach to changeover for Y and Z, then there will be a large amount of testing required since changeovers occur once per week. If it wants to adopt a validation approach to changeover for products Y and Z, meetings will have to be reconvened and documents will have to be revised to describe an additional approach to changeover. A great deal of this revisiting effort could have been saved if Company GHI had made the initial descriptions of its changeover approach flexible enough to cover both verification and validation.

In summary, the changeover program in a multiproduct biotechnology facility can take several forms, including verification, validation, or a combination of both. The choice of method depends largely upon the characteristics of the process and the frequency of changeovers. Regardless of which method is chosen, a resource investment must be made to initiate and maintain the program. In addition, sufficient thought must be put into program development to ensure that the program can be applied to all of the company's products.

EQUIPMENT CONSIDERATIONS

The choice of equipment for a multiproduct facility is an important element in how well the facility will function. The equipment can be broken down into three major categories: processing equipment, raw material preparation/transfer/storage equipment, and cleaning equipment. This section will address the issue of equipment dedication, and then conclude with a discussion of issues related to each of the three categories of equipment described above.

Equipment: Dedicated or Non-Dedicated?

When choosing equipment for a multiproduct facility, the choice must be made between the use of dedicated equipment, non-dedicated equipment, or a combination of both. In the case of work with spore-bearing organisms, one must use dedicated equipment [4], but for other products, this decision is typically made by weighing a number of factors. Table 8.1, below, provides a list of some of these factors, along with a judgement about whether each factor is a plus or a minus in the decision to dedicate. Generally, these factors will be weighed and the decision of whether to dedicate equipment will be made by balancing the cost of dedication versus the cost of changeover.

By reviewing Table 8.1, one can see that there are several benefits of choosing dedicated equipment. The potential for cross contamination from the equipment is eliminated, provided that the dedicated items are properly labeled and segregated. The complexity of the cleaning validation program is reduced.

Table 8.1
Dedicated vs. Non-Dedicated Equipment in a Multiproduct Facility

Issue	Dedicated Equipment	Non-Dedicated Equipment
1. Potential for cross contamination from equipment	no (+)	yes (−)
2. Capital investment in equipment for each product	high (−)	low (+)
3. Complexity of cleaning validation program	low (+)	high (−)
4. Time required to changeover a production area	long (−)	short (+)
5. Storage space requirements	high (−)	low (+)
6. Complexity of equipment (flexible equipment design required?)	no (+)	yes (−)
7. Equipment qualifications (IQs and OQs)	many (−)	few (+)

The potential for cross contamination is eliminated because new equipment is purchased for each product. The cleaning validation program is simpler because there is no need for a changeover element. The primary goal of the program, then, shifts from preventing cross contamination between products to preventing cross contamination between batches.

Using dedicated equipment also has its drawbacks. The purchase of new equipment for each product is expensive, especially such large/installed items as fermentors and process piping. Additionally, sufficient storage space must be available to store the dedicated equipment when another product is in the production area. Finally, the use of dedicated processing equipment can increase the time necessary for product changeover because, at the end of the campaign, the dedicated equipment is typically removed from the production area and replaced with the equipment for the next process.

As with dedicated equipment, there are several benefits associated with the use of non-dedicated equipment. Capital is saved because new equipment does not have to be purchased for each product. The savings from the use of non-dedicated equipment are not only the monetary savings resulting from a reduced number of equipment purchases, but also both the time and monetary savings resulting from not having to perform initial qualifications (IQs and OQs) for many sets of dedicated equipment.

There are several drawbacks to the use of non-dedicated equipment. If the equipment is not cleaned properly, there is the potential for cross contamination. The cleaning validation program now becomes more complex because it must include a changeover element. Finally, the equipment must be designed with the flexibility to produce multiple products. For example, a filling line must be designed to fill a large number of different sizes and types of vials.

As mentioned previously, it is possible to choose equipment that has a combination of dedicated and non-dedicated parts. An example would be an ultrafiltration skid where the piping and controls are nondedicated and the filter membranes are dedicated. The choice of combination equipment such as this allows one to get the cost advantages of non-dedicated equipment without the problems of changeover associated with the more complex elements of the system.

Another approach that can be taken is to dedicate equipment until it becomes cost effective to perform the cleaning validation studies necessary to make a dedicated item non-dedicated. This approach can allow a company to delay the resource investment required for changeover. In this way, the decision to dedicate something is reversible.

In summary, there are many issues to be considered when deciding between dedicated and non-dedicated equipment. Choosing dedicated equipment is attractive because its choice minimizes the possibility of cross contamination and simplifies the cleaning validation effort. Choosing non-dedicated equipment is attractive because its choice offers capital efficiency, allows for faster changeovers, and requires minimal storage space. One can also choose combination equipment, which has some of the benefits of both dedicated and non-dedicated equipment. Finally, the decision to dedicate something can be reversed if it becomes economically desirable.

Processing Equipment Considerations

There are several factors that can make the use of processing equipment easier in a multiproduct facility. These include flexibility of design and equipment with replaceable product contact surfaces. In addition, the use of disposable items can simplify the cleaning validation effort. However, there are some items that are typically product-dedicated due to the difficulties associated with validating their cleaning.

Due to the cost and installation/validation time required for certain types of equipment (e.g., fermentors, filling lines), these items are typically non-dedicated in a multiproduct facility. To get maximum use out of these types of non-dedicated equipment, they should be designed with flexibility in mind. It might be difficult during the design of the first multiproduct plant to envision all of the potential products that might be manufactured there. However, time spent up front in the planning is well worth the effort several years down the line. For example, tanks for cell culture can be designed so that they are adaptable to either microbial or mammalian cells. Chromatography columns can be ordered with adjustable flow adapter bore sizes to allow for a wide range of flow rates.

Other options that should be considered when choosing processing equipment for a multiproduct facility are the use of disposable items and items with replaceable product contact surfaces. With disposables, there is no risk of cross contamination, but the added cost of replenishment and the need for adequate storage space are drawbacks. Equipment with replaceable product contact surfaces (e.g., peristaltic pumps) is ideal; however there are very few types of equipment like this available.

Finally, there are some items that are usually dedicated to a specific product due to the difficulty of assuring that they are clean. The difficulty typically arises from the fact that items like resins, membranes, and filters have a large surface area that is not easily accessible to non-destructive testing. However, the decision of which items to dedicate must be left up to individual manufacturers, since they best know the effort required to validate the cleaning of each piece of equipment.

In summary, there are several issues to be considered when choosing processing equipment for a multiproduct facility. These issues include: flexibility of design, disposable equipment, and equipment with replaceable product contact surfaces. There are also some types of equipment that are typically dedicated due to the difficulty associated with validating their cleanliness.

Raw Material Preparation/Transfer/Storage Equipment Considerations

In a multiproduct facility, there is generally a category of equipment that is non-dedicated, but that does not contact product directly. This equipment typically consists of raw material preparation vessels, solution transfer piping, and media and buffer storage vessels. While the risk of cross contamination of products is not a concern with this equipment, cleaning must still be validated due to the possibility of cross contamination of raw materials. This possibility is greatest in a concurrent manufacturing scenario, where multiple products are being produced simultaneously.

Cross contamination may be a concern because a specific process may not be able to remove the raw materials used in other processes. The degree of concern about raw material cross contamination depends largely on the characteristics of the raw materials utilized. Oftentimes, the raw materials used for any given product are not significantly different from the raw materials used for any other product. In some cases, however, a specific process has a raw material that may pose more of a risk if cross contamination occurs. If such a raw material is identified, special evaluation should be conducted to determine if additional cleaning studies or equipment dedication is necessary.

When designing a cleaning validation program for non-dedicated preparation, transfer, or storage equipment, the number and type of raw materials utilized should be considered. Since a large number of solutions are prepared, transferred, and stored in this type of equipment, a bracketing approach to cleaning validation is typically utilized. The test solutions used in the validation study should represent the worst case in terms of concentration and type of raw materials used. For example, in a buffer preparation area, the test solution could be the most concentrated salt and surfactant containing buffer prepared; and in a media preparation area, the test solution could be the media with the highest protein concentration.

The bracketing approach described above is the start to a good basic cleaning validation program for multiproduct raw material preparation/transfer/storage equipment. However, the cleaning validation program for these items must be an ongoing effort if the multiproduct facility is continually using new raw materials. The ongoing effort is required to evaluate the raw materials of each new process against the existing cleaning validations done for the preparation, transfer, and storage equipment. As mentioned above, if a raw material is identified that poses a special concern, a decision must be made with regard to additional studies or equipment dedication.

To sum up, cleaning validation must be performed on raw material preparation/transfer/ storage equipment to minimize the risk of cross contamination of raw materials. For these types of vessels and piping, a bracketing approach to cleaning validation is typically utilized. Finally, if the facility is continually using new raw materials, an ongoing effort must be maintained to assess the impact of the new raw materials on the existing cleaning validation studies.

Cleaning Equipment Considerations

In a multiproduct facility, in addition to non-dedicated processing and raw material preparation/storage/transfer equipment, there is also typically non-dedicated cleaning equipment. This equipment can include clean-in-place (CIP) systems, glassware washers, and parts washers. The risk of cross contamination from cleaning equipment is due to the possibility that product could be left in the cleaning equipment following the cleaning cycle, and that it could be released into the next cleaning cycle. As with preparation, transfer, and storage equipment, the risk of cross contamination from cleaning equipment is greatest in the concurrent manufacturing scenario.

Like processing equipment, there are some cleaning equipment design elements that can minimize or eliminate the potential for cross contamination from the cleaning equipment. For example, a central plant CIP system that serves multiple production areas can be designed to be non-recirculating. If no solutions return to the CIP system, then the possibility of cross contamination is eliminated. Another alternative is a central CIP system that only supplies the cleaning solutions and rinses to the equipment. Separate circulation pumps can then be used to recirculate the cleaning solutions. This approach saves water, but involves a more complex CIP system. Still another approach is a separate CIP system for each production area. This approach minimizes cross contamination, but is more costly initially, and requires more time to validate multiple CIP systems.

Regardless of what type of CIP system is chosen, there are several design elements that can maximize the utility of the system in a multiproduct environment. Some of these include:

- The system should be able to supply a variety of flow rates (through the use of a variable speed pump or a throttling valve).

- Flowmeters should have the widest range of flow rates possible. If the flowmeter range is not broad, the system should be designed so that the flowmeter can easily be replaced with one of a different range.

- The alarm setpoints should be programmable, and not factory set.

- The chemical addition equipment should be able to handle a range of chemicals.

- The cleaning step sequence should be programmable on site.

In facilities where more than one production area utilize a shared glasswash or equipment clean-out-of-place (COP) area, cross contamination concerns must be addressed. In addition to an appropriate labeling system to segregate equipment, the glassware and parts washers should be examined for potential areas of concern. If these items are used to clean product contact equipment from different products, then they are potential sites for cross contamination.

These concerns can be minimized by running loads dedicated to a single product, minimizing hold-over of water between loads, and restricting product contact items from the glassware and parts washers. If product contact items are washed in the glassware or parts washer, the cleaning cycles must be validated to ensure that product is not carried from one load to the next.

In summary, many multiproduct facilities utilize non-dedicated cleaning equipment. To get the maximum use out of these pieces of cleaning equipment, they should be designed with flexibility in mind. There are also certain modes of operation (e.g., non-recirculation, minimum water hold-over) that can minimize the potential for cross contamination.

SUMMARY

Cleaning validation is essential for the licensure of multiproduct biotechnology production facilities. Multiproduct facilities are becoming more common today as manufacturers look to reduce the cost, risk, and time to bring new drugs to market. Multiproduct facilities are particularly attractive as their use allows a company to spread the initial facility investment over several products.

The primary difference between a cleaning validation program in a dedicated versus a multiproduct facility is the requirement for a changeover element in a multiproduct facility's program. This element can take the form of validation, verification, or a combination of both. Whichever approach is selected, the goal of the changeover element is to demonstrate that equipment has been adequately cleaned to ensure fitness for use in the next production process.

When equipment is purchased for use in a multiproduct facility, the choice must be made between dedicated and non-dedicated equipment. There are benefits and drawbacks to both choices. The decision typically comes down to an analysis of whether it is cheaper to buy new equipment for each product or to perform the necessary changeover cleaning validation studies.

A multiproduct facility typically has a variety of non-dedicated equipment—including processing equipment, raw material preparation/transfer/storage equipment, and cleaning equipment. To get the maximum use out of each piece of non-dedicated equipment, flexible design of the equipment is critical. For raw material preparation/transfer/storage equipment, a bracketing approach to cleaning validation is typically utilized. One must be sure, however, to have a system in place for evaluating new raw materials against existing cleaning validation studies.

In conclusion, the use of multiproduct facilities can be attractive, but the issues associated with changeover are not insignificant. With well designed equipment and a sound changeover cleaning validation strategy, a multiproduct biotechnology manufacturing facility can be extremely successful.

REFERENCES

1. Hill, D. and Beatrice, M., "Facility Requirements for Biotech Plants," *Pharmaceutical Engineering,* 9(4), 1989, pp 35–41.

2. Bader, et al., "Multiuse Manufacturing Facilities for Biologicals," *BioPharm*, 5(7), 1992, pp 32–40.

3. Personal communication, H. Michael Koplove, Vice-President of Manufacturing Operations and Process Technology, Genetics Institute, 1992.

4. Code of Federal Regulations, Title 21, Parts 600–800. Revised April 1, 1991.

5. Code of Federal Regulations, Title 21, Parts 200–211. Revised April 1, 1991.

6. Avallone, H., "GMP Inspections of Biopharmaceutical Manufacturing Facilities," *Pharmaceutical Engineering*, 9(5), 1989, pp 40–48.

7. Hill, D., and Beatrice, M., "Biotechnology Facility Requirements, Part II: Operating Procedures and Validation," *BioPharm* 2 (10), 1989, pp 28–31.

8. DelCiello, R., and Snell, J., "Economics of Current Good Manufacturing Practice Design," *Pharmaceutical Engineering,* 6(2), 1986, pp 32–51.

9. Rosenburg, R., "Growing Biotech Industry Facing New Pressures from Health Care Reform, Lack of Financing," *Boston Globe*, March 7, 1993.

10. Bisbee, C.A., "Experts Discuss Strategies to Finance Biomanufacturing," *Genetic Engineering News,* 14(9), 1994, pp 1–34.

11. Agarwal, D., et al., "Design Concepts for Multipurpose Bulk Pharmaceutical Facilities," *Pharmaceutical Engineering,* 10(1), 1990, pp 27–31.

Glossary

Campaign Manufacturing: Processing of more than one product in the same facility and/or equipment in a sequential manner. Only one product is present in any one manufacturing area of the facility at a time.

Changeover: The process of preparing a piece of equipment used for the production of a specific product for the production of a different product. Changeover usually includes cleaning, sampling, and testing to assure fitness for use in the next production process.

Combination Approach: The combination approach is the use of the verification approach until sufficient repeats of the cleaning procedure have been performed to consider the cleaning procedure validated.

Concurrent Manufacturing: Concurrent manufacturing in a multiproduct facility is characterized by simultaneous production of a number of different products in segregated areas within the same facility.

Dedicated Equipment: Equipment that is permanently used for the production of only one product.

Multiproduct Facility: Manufacturing facility that contains areas for the processing of two or more products either concurrently or on a campaigned basis.

Non-Dedicated Equipment: Equipment that is used for the production of more than one product.

Verification Approach: Verification is the process of sampling and testing to ensure that a piece of equipment has been properly cleaned following *each* use.

Appendix

Process Validation of the Cleaning and Changeover Procedure for Process Tank T-XXXX

A. INTRODUCTION

System XXX.X, the Process tank (T-XXXX), is used in the production of Bulk product. The system contains a chilled glycol heat transfer system to maintain operating temperatures. A bottom mounted agitator provides mixing during processing. Following use, the tank and associated piping are cleaned using the Clean-in-Place (CIP) System (System XXX). Before initiating a new product campaign, the process tank is partially disassembled and cleaned per an established changeover procedure. This changeover procedure is designed to prevent possible cross-contamination of various products previously processed in the tank. Following changeover procedures, the tank is reassembled and again cleaned by CIP to provide further assurance of cleanliness.

B. PURPOSE

This protocol is designed to evaluate the effectiveness of the cleaning and changeover process for the Process tank (T-XXXX). This study shall confirm that the cleaning and changeover process, performed according to a standard operating procedure, is reliable and in a state of control.

C. SCOPE

Standard operating procedure SOPXXXXX is used for changeover of the Process tank (T–XXXX). Following a production run, the tank is cleaned per SOPXXXXX. Final rinse samples are collected from the cleaned equipment. These samples are tested for pH (AMXXX) and conductivity (AMXXX) using SDS-PAGE with silver stain (AMXXX), a product-specific immunoassay (per appropriate analytical method) and total organic carbon (AMXXX). These samples are also tested for LAL (AMXXX) and Total Aerobic Microbial Count (SOPXXXXX) to determine endotoxin and bioburden levels. This testing is designed to demonstrate effective removal of product residues and cleaning residues.

Prior to initiating a new product campaign in the Process tank, a changeover procedure must take place. Changeover involves some disassembly and cleaning of tank components. At the beginning and end of the changeover process, representative product-contact surfaces are sampled and tested for total organic carbon (AMXXX). This testing is designed to determine the level of residual product/contaminant from the previous campaign.

After surface sampling, the equipment is reassembled and recleaned per SOPXXXX. Final rinse samples again are collected from the cleaned equipment. These samples are tested for pH (AMXXX) and conductivity (AMXXX) using SDS-PAGE with silver stain (AMXXX), a product-specific immunoassay (per appropriate analytical method), total organic carbon (AMXXX), LAL (AMXXX), and total aerobic microbial count (SOPXXXX) as before. This testing is designed to demonstrate that no additional contaminants have been introduced into the system as a result of the changeover procedure.

D. REFERENCES

1. Standard Operating Procedure
    1.1 SOPXXXX: Changeover Cleaning Procedure for the Process tank (T-XXXX)
    1.2 SOPXXXX: Cleaning Procedure for the Process tank (T-XXXX)
    1.3 SOPXXXX: Total Aerobic Microbial Count

2. Analytical Methods
    2.1 AMXXX: LAL Test for the Determination of Bacterial Endotoxin Content of Solutions
    2.2 AMXXX: Conductivity Measurement
    2.3 AMXXX: Total Organic Carbon Analysis

2.4   AMXXX: pH Determination

2.5   AMXXX: SDS-PAGE with Silver Staining

2.6   AMXXX: Product X, specific enzyme immunoassay

2.7   AMXXX: Product Y, radioreceptor assay

3.   Validation Documents

3.1   XXX-PV-XXX: Process Validation: Cleaning of Process tank T-XXXX

3.2   VP-X-XX: Validation Policy: Surface Sampling for Total Organic Carbon

E.   EQUIPMENT AND MATERIALS

1.   Review documents listed in Section D, References, for other appropriate equipment

2.   Process tank (T-XXXX)

3.   Appropriately sized sterile sample containers

4.   Surface sampling kits

F.   RESPONSIBILITIES

1.   Validation

1.1   Protocol generation, review, and approval

1.2   Perform all surface sampling which corresponds to this protocol

1.3   Assist manufacturing personnel with final rinse samples as appropriate

1.4   Data review and acceptance

1.5   Final report review and approval

1.6   Scheduling validation and revalidation

2.   Production

2.1   Protocol review and approval

2.2   Perform all final rinse aseptic sampling which corresponds to this protocol

2.3   Data review and acceptance

2.4   Final report completeness and applicability

2.5   Final report generation, review, and approval

3.   Process Maintenance

3.1   Perform disassembly and reassembly as required by the changeover procedure

4.   Quality Control/Analytical Resources

4.1   Protocol review and approval

4.2   Conduct appropriate assays and report results on a timely basis

4.3   Final report review and approval

5. Quality Assurance Microbiology
    5.1 Protocol review and approval
    5.2 Conduct appropriate assays and report results on a timely basis
    5.3 Final report review and approval

6. Quality Assurance
    6.1 Protocol review and approval
    6.2 Final report review and approval

G. TEST PROCEDURE

1. Rinse Sample Collection
    1.1 Set-up the sample collection pump and attach tubing to the drain port on the CIP return pump. Exact location and configuration will be diagrammed in the final report.
    1.2 Flush sample tubing continuously for the duration of the CIP cycle.This ensures that the sample tubing is exposed to the same types of chemicals and rinses that the process equipment is exposed to during CIP. Flushing should provide an accurate sample representation from the sample tubing.
    1.3 Distribute all samples as indicated in Section G, step 6.

2. Post-Campaign Cleaning: Process tank (T-XXXX)
    2.1 Following a normal formulation/filtration run, perform the cleaning procedure on the Process tank (T-XXXX) per SOPXXXX. In addition, the tank may be dirtied using the procedure described in Appendix A.
    2.2 At the beginning of the pre-rinse cycle, aseptically collect one (1) one-liter WFI pre-rinse sample. Label sample as "T-XXXX Post-Campaign Cleaning—Pre-Rinse." Sample collection set-up is detailed in Section G, step 1.
    2.3 At the end of the recirculation cycle, aseptically collect one (1)-liter WFI final rinse sample. Label sample as "T-XXXX Post-Campaign Cleaning—Recirculation Final Rinse." Sample collection set-up is detailed in Section G, step 1.
    2.4 Monitor the conductivity meter on the CIP control panel. When the display reads ≤ 40 μS, aseptically collect one (1) one-liter WFI final rinse sample. Label sample as "T-XXXX Post-Campaign Cleaning—Middle Final Rinse." Sample collection set-up is detailed in Section G, step 1.
    2.5 At the end of the final rinse cycle (conductivity display on the CIP control panel reads < 25 μS), aseptically collect one (1) one-liter WFI final rinse sample. Label sample as "T-XXXX Post-

Run Cleaning—End Final Rinse." Sample collection set-up is detailed in Section G, step 1.

3. Changeover: Process tank (T-XXXX)

   3.1 Disassemble the Process tank (T-XXXX) per changeover procedure SOPXXXX. Make sure the equipment has been cleaned per the appropriate SOP prior to changeover. Record visual observations of the sites to be sampled by on a copy of Table 1.

   3.2 Following disassembly but prior to cleaning, perform surface sampling per VP-X-XXX at the locations described in Diagram 1.

   3.3 Clean Process tank (T-XXXX) components per changeover procedure SOPXXXX. If components are cleaned in the COP bath, aseptically collect a one (1) one-liter final rinse WFI sample from the COP bath drain valve. Label sample as "T-XXXX Component COP—Final Rinse."

   3.4 After cleaning but prior to reassembly, perform surface sampling again per VP-X-XXX at the locations described in Diagram 1. This sampling should mimic the sampling that was performed in Section G, step 3.2.

   3.5 After surface sampling, reassemble the Process tank (T-XXXX) per changeover procedure SOPXXXX.

4. Post-Changeover Cleaning: Process tank (T-XXXX)

   4.1 Perform the cleaning procedure on Process tank (T-XXXX) per SOPXXXX. Make sure the equipment has undergone changeover per the appropriate SOP prior to cleaning.

   4.2 At the beginning of the pre-rinse cycle, aseptically collect one (1) one-liter WFI pre-rinse sample. Label sample as "T-XXXX Post-Changeover Cleaning—Pre-Rinse." Sample collection set-up is detailed in Section G, step 1.

   4.3 At the end of the recirculation cycle, aseptically collect one (1) one-liter WFI final rinse sample. Label sample as "T-XXXX Post–Changeover Cleaning—Recirculation Final Rinse." Sample collection set-up is detailed in Section G, step 1.

   4.4 Monitor the conductivity meter on the CIP control panel. When the display reads ≤ 40 µS, aseptically collect one (1) one-liter WFI final rinse sample. Label sample as "T-XXXX Post-Changeover Cleaning—Middle Final Rinse." Sample collection set-up is detailed in Section G, step 1.

   4.5 At the end of the final rinse cycle (conductivity display on the CIP control panel reads < 25 µS), aseptically collect one (1) one-Liter WFI final rinse sample. Label sample as "T-XXXX Post-

Changeover Cleaning—End Final Rinse." Sample collection set-up is detailed in Section G, step 1.

5. Data Acquisition
    5.1 All data that pertain to this protocol must be recorded. This information can be included in the final report as raw data.

6. Sample Distribution
    6.1 Aseptically aliquot the 1 x 1 liter final rinse WFI samples as follows:
        6.1.1 1 x 200 ml into a sterile polystyrene bottle for both pH determination per USP and conductivity analysis per AM-XXX. Affix pre-printed label and submit to lab for testing.
        6.1.2 1 x 50 ml into a sterile glass bottle for total organic carbon analysis per AMXXX. Affix pre-printed labels and submit to lab for testing.
        6.1.3 1 x 50 ml into a sterile polypropylene sample tube for SDS-PAGE with Silver Staining per AMXXX. Affix pre-printed label and submit to lab for testing.
        6.1.4 1 x 20 ml into a sterile polypropylene sample tube for product-specific assay testing per the appropriate procedure. This testing should be for the product that was *previously* prepared in the equipment. Affix pre-printed label and submit to lab for testing.
        6.1.5 1 x 15 ml into a sterile polystyrene sample tube for LAL testing per AMXXX. Affix pre-printed label and submit to Microbiology for testing.
        6.1.6 1 x 250 ml into a sterile polypropylene container for Total Aerobic Microbial Count analysis per SOPXXXX. Affix pre-printed label and submit to Microbiology for testing.
        6.1.7 Keep the remainder of the 1 x 1 *l* sample of the WFI flush for reserve. Affix a pre-printed label and store reserve sample at $5 \pm 3°C$.
    6.2 Surface samples are collected into 50 ml glass tubes for total organic carbon per AMXXX. Affix pre-printed labels and submit to lab for testing.

7. Assays
    7.1 The following assays are to be performed. Results are to be recorded on appropriate forms and data are to be included in final report.

TITLE	ASSAY NO.	VOLUME/CONTAINER
pH Determination	USP	200 ml/polystyrene
Conductivity	ANXXX	(from pH sample)
Total Organic Carbon	ANXXX	50 ml/glass
SDS-Page with Ag+ stain	ANXXX	50 ml/polypropylene
Product Specific Assay	ANXXX	20 ml/polypropylene
LAL	ANXXX	15 ml/polystyrene
Total Aerobic Microbial Count (TAMC)	SOPXXXX	250 ml polypropylene (100 ml TO BE PLATED)

8. Acceptance Criteria

   8.1 Three successful validation runs for each changeover operation in which the samples meet the following criteria constitutes successful completion of this protocol:

     (Note: FIO = For Information Only)

     8.1.1   Post-Campaign Cleaning Final Rinse Samples

Sample Description	pH (ANXX)	Cond. (ANXX)	TOC (AMXX)	SDS-PAGE (ANXX)	Prod Specific (AMXX)	LAL (AMXX)	TAMC (ANXX)
Pre-Rinse	FIO	FIO	FIO	FIO	FIO	FIO	FIO
Recirc.	FIO	FIO	FIO	FIO	FIO	FIO	FIO
Middle	FIO	FIO	FIO	FIO	FIO	FIO	FIO
End	5.0–7.0 25 ± 2°C	<20 µS/cm 25 ± 2°C	≤ 1 ppm	No detectable contam.	< 1 ppm	≤ 2.5 Eu/ml	FIO

     8.1.2   Changeover Surface Samples

Sample Description	TOC (ANXXX)
All	≤ 1 ppm

     8.1.3   Component COP Final Rinse Samples

Sample Description	pH (ANXX)	Cond. (ANXX)	TOC (AMXX)	SDS-PAGE (ANXX)	Prod Specific	LAL (AMXX)	TAMC (ANXX)
Final Rinse	5.0–7.0 25 ± 2°C	<20 µS/cm 25 ± 2°C	≤ 1 ppm	No detectable contam.	< 1 ppm	≤ 2.5 Eu/ml	FIO

8.1.4 Post-Changeover Cleaning Final Rinse Samples

Sample Description	pH (ANXX)	Cond. (ANXX)	TOC (AMXX)	SDS-PAGE (ANXX)	Prod Specific	LAL (AMXX)	TAMC (ANXX)
Pre-Rinse	FIO	FIO	FIO	FIO	FIO	FIO	FIO
Recirc.	FIO	FIO	FIO	FIO	FIO	FIO	FIO
Middle	FIO	FIO	FIO	FIO	FIO	FIO	FIO
End	5.0–7.0 25 ± 2°C	<20 µS/cm 25 ± 2°C	≤ 1 ppm	No detectable contam.	< 1 ppm	≤ 2.5 Eu/ml	FIO

Table 1
RUN # _____   Pre- or Post-Cleaning (circle one)

Sample	Sample Description	Observations	Initial/Date
01	SIGHT GLASS (2" x 2")		
02	VENT FILTER PORT		
03	MANWAY FLANGE		
04	TOP DOME INTERIOR (2" x 2")		
05	2" PORT INTERIOR SURFACE		
06	MIDDLE PLANE-MANWAY (2" x 2")		
07	MIDDLE PLANE-VENT PORT (2" x 2")		
08	MIDDLE PLANE-BACK (2" x 2")		
09	MIDDLE PLANE-OPPOSITE AGITATOR (2" x 2")		
10	BOTTOM PLANE-MANWAY (2" x 2")		
11	BOTTOM PLANE-VENT PORT (2" x 2")		
12	BOTTOM PLANE-BACK (2" x 2")		
13	BOTTOM PLANE-OPP. AGITATOR (2" x 2")		
14	IMPELLER SURFACE (2" x 2")		
15	IMPELLER BUSHING		
16	DRAIN PORT		
17	MANWAY GASKET		
18	DRAIN VALVE DIAPHRAGM		

Index

absorbance scans, 123
acceptance criteria, 92, 97, 100, 113,
    129–142
acceptance limits, 131–141
acidic cleaners, 45–47, 56, 59–61
agents, cleaning, 34–35, 41–51, 54,
    58–63, 69, 78, 80, 83–85, 92, 96,
    98–99, 101, 105, 110, 115, 118,
    125, 139–140
agitators, 22, 25, 27
air detection, 34
alkaline cleaners, 44–46, 50, 54–55, 86
analytical methods, specific, 99, 117
analytical methods, non-specific, 117
anionic wetting agents, 46–47
assays, specific, 117–118, 120–122,
    126–127, 137
assays, non-specific, 123–126

baffles, 22, 26–27
balance, hydraulically, 15
BCA method, 124
biological contaminants, 98, 119–120
bioreactors, 3, 5–9, 108
biowaste systems, 36
Biuret method, 124

BL1 organisms, 4
BL3 cell culture process, 6
Bradford method, 124
bracketing, 156–158
breakers, vortex, 22, 23, 27

calcium, 44–45, 47
calibration verification, 94
campaigned basis of production, 147,
    149–150, 161
cation, 44, 46–47
centralized utilities, 147
centrifuges, 36–37
changeover, 36, 117, 120, 123,
    148–155, 158, 161
chaotropic agents, 119
chelants, 44, 46
chemical erosion, 49–51, 82
chlorine, 45–46, 58, 61
chromatography systems, 31, 60–62,
    139
chromatography columns, 3, 28, 35,
    60–61, 155
CIP. *See* clean-in-place
circuits, 4–5, 9, 15, 17, 19, 51, 71, 80,
    95, 109